MW01069948

No Fricken

Weigh!

21 Days to Ditch the Diet, Lose Weight the Keto Way, By Loving Yourself to Health

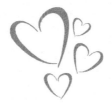

By Tracee Gluhaich, CHHC, CPT aka the High Energy Girl

All rights reserved. No part of this book may be reproduced, scanned, or distributed in any printed or electronic form without permission in writing from the author. Please do not participate in or encourage piracy of copyrighted materials in violation of the authors' rights. Purchase only authorized editions. No patent liability is assumed with respect to the use of the information contained herein. Although every precaution has been taken in the preparation of this book, the publisher and the author assume no responsibility for errors or omissions. Neither is any liability assumed for damages resulting from the use of information contained herein. These statements have not been evaluated by the FDA and are not intended to diagnose, treat, cure, or prevent disease.

This publication contains the opinion and thoughts of the author. It is intended to provide helpful and informative material on the subjects covered. It is sold with the understanding that the author and publisher are not engaged in rendering professional services in the book. If the reader requires personal assistance or advice a competent professional should be consulted.

The authors and publisher specifically disclaim any responsibility for any liability, loss, or risk, personal or otherwise, which is incurred as a consequence, directly or indirectly, of the use and application of any of the contents of this book.

Copyright © 2019 by Tracee Gluhaich

Printed in the United States of America

FREE BONUSES

Find all the free bonuses on the page below. There is a health checklist, cookbook, guides, meal plans and special webinar trainings. There may even be an audio book in the future!

These bonuses will be updated as time goes on and you will have special promos and access to coaching. Claim these right away.

Grab all bonuses here: http://HighEnergyGirl.com/nfwbonus

I am here to support you in aging stronger.You are not too old and it's never too late.

Namaste!

PS Don't forget to join my Facebook Group: High Energy Girls

Acknowledgements

This book would not be possible without patience and love from many people. I would like to thank God for saving me through my tumultuous years, so I can serve the purpose He chose for my life.

Thank you to my wonderful hubby, Pete, for incredible patience and for loving me for the last 30 years.

Thanks to my awesome boys, I mean men, Marko, Nick, and David, for giving me the inspiration to make myself a better person and for giving me the gift of motherhood.

Big hugs to my mom and mother-in-law, my 2 best cheerleaders.

Thanks to Roxy for your daily support.

Thank you to all the girls at High Energy Girl for keeping me inspired.

NO FRICKEN WEIGH!

NO FRICKEN WEIGH!

Introduction

This is NOT a Diet Book.

This is NOT a Fitness Book.

This is a Hope Book.

With the thousands of books on the market teaching us to improve our health, everyone should be thin, fit and happy. But instead, our country is full of fat, sick, and depressed couch potatoes. It doesn't have to be this way.

There is something missing, something that keeps us from applying what we should already know. The purpose of this book is to close the gap.

If you ever:

- experienced an energy crash
- deprived yourself on a diet
- looked in the mirror and hated the reflection
- felt weak, old, fluffy, or unhappy

then this book is for you!

You are probably wondering how this book is going to help you and why it is different than all of the other 307,549 "health books" sold online.

What this book is going to teach you is how to ditch the traditional diet mentality of deprivation, and how you can heal your body with self-care and nourishing foods.

We talk about how you can reduce inflammation, literally age stronger, turn back the hands of time, and become the best version of yourself possible.

Instead of going on a diet and killing yourself in the gym, you will learn to eat life building foods to help your body thrive and increase your energy. You will build your metabolism and grow stronger. Your body will become shapelier and you will feel sexier.

Since many experts say that it takes 21 days to adopt a new habit, I'm including 21 ways to fill your life with joy and 21 fantastic foods to strengthen your body.

Sprinkled throughout the book are motivational quotes, in no particular order. I just LOVE a good quote to chew on every day and hope they inspire you as well!

There are a few writing challenges scattered throughout the book as well. So, purchase a journal to keep all your writing together. And do yourself a favor, take a break, put the book down and complete the exercises.

Are you ready to transform? Turn the page and let's get started.

PART 1

WHY ARE YOU FLUFFY?

My Passion and Purpose in Writing This Book

When I was 10 years old, my Dad came home with a bad ass brand-new yellow Rally Sport Camaro. He ran upstairs and came down with a suitcase. He told me, "Tell your mom I am leaving." I was startled and confused. Mom came home, I told her what he had said, and she shared the horrifying details.

Four months later, he married the skinny b$%#@, that he had been cheating with, and took on a whole new family. His new wife had a beautiful daughter, who I was insanely jealous of, and a son. My younger brother and I were kicked to the curb and I felt abandoned.

A short time later, I remembered an argument that my parents had, when my dad said, to my mom, "If you ever get fat again, I am leaving you." Which he did! So, I put two and two together (cuz I can add) and the message to my 10-year-old self was skinny = love.

So, my quest for skinny and the dieting obsession began. Now mind you, I was never really that overweight, maybe 10 lbs. or so. I was a curvy Italianish (because I am only ¼ but I took on that appearance) girl surrounded by skinny friends.

It started with the Cambridge Diet, then Beverly Hills, then Diet Center, and continued. The summer before my sophomore year in high school, I went on the iced tea diet, which I totally made up. Basically, I was starving myself and only drinking iced tea to get an energy hit from the caffeine. I must have drunk a gallon of sun tea a day.

When I showed up to the first day of school, looking skinny (and hot), everyone complimented me on how great I looked; I was so excited. Once again equating skinny with love.

By the time I was in college, I had been on every type of diet imaginable, continuously striving for skinny and searching for love and acceptance. I alternated periods of starving and the rebound bingeing.

Then the high impact aerobics craze started, it was the 80's you know! Wink! So, I jumped on in. Since I am pigeon-toed and bow legged, I got horrible shin splints and thought I was going to die. Since, I was so obsessed with my mission, I would take Advil an hour before my aerobics class and I wouldn't feel any pain...until the medication wore off and I could hardly stand.

Fast forward 5 years, I graduated from college and met my future husband. I finally found true love and thought my turmoil would end. And it did for a while.

When I was thinking about getting pregnant, the obsession with skinny transferred to wanting to be the healthiest mom possible. The demon kindly disappeared. Years later, it resurfaced, popping in and out of my life when I was not expecting it. The bastard! My obsession with skinny was back and forth as I raised my children.

Finally, in 2007, I started studying nutrition. I really wanted to break the pattern and raise healthy kids. I wanted to help them establish better eating habits then I had.

My youngest was already 10, and I had raised them on the typical kid cuisine of chicken nuggets, PB&J, frozen pizza, mac n cheese, and corn dogs. So, I had a whole hell of a lot of retraining to do.

My personal focus was starting to change from the number on the scale, to being a healthy mom and raising healthy humans.

During my schooling, I pondered why both my parents had numerous degenerative diseases at young ages. My mom had Alzheimer's and Hashimoto's. And my dad had a heart attack and cancer four times. They have both been taking multiple medications for as long as I can remember. So, my genes are really stacked against me.

In nutrition school, I learned that food can be our medicine. I was super excited to learn about the power of food and I really wanted to help both of my parents with their diseases.

So, I did some self-study and tons of research on nutritional protocols to heal their bodies and tackle the root cause of their diseases. I listened to podcasts, read books and watched documentaries, searching for an answer to help my parents figure out a natural solution.

This research really shifted my thinking and made me determined to NOT age in sickness, but in health. I also learned a harsh reality. You can lead a horse to water, but you can't make them drink. Sadly, neither of my parents were a thirsty horse.

So, with all my research, what did I learn?

In 1958, a researcher, who shall not be named, published the Seven Countries Study. He hypothesized that a diet high in fat increased the risk of heart disease. However, for some strange and mysterious reason, the data from 15 other countries, that didn't align with his hypothesis, were not included. He is definitely one of the pricks, steamrolling our country for all of these decades.

However, nobody else smelled that stinky fish and our country went on a decades long, fat-free obsession.

What do you think happened to our waistlines during this time? The obesity rate increased substantially, and Americans got sicker.

We were essentially lied to. We were told that fat made us fat and was the evil emperor, the arch enemy. So, we ditched the fat and in order to still have flavor, the food manufacturers replaced it with sugar.

> We believe it is possible to age healthier and stronger. The way we challenge the current aging dogma is by creating strong bodies and smart minds. We provide help and coaching every step of the way. Ready to get started? ~High Energy Girl

All this time, I thought I was eating healthy. I was living off of fat free everything: bagels, potatoes, refried beans, cheese and tortillas. Do you know how bad fat-free cheese tastes? OMG cannot believe I fell for that load of crap. These "foods" didn't taste great, but since they were fat free, they must have been good for me, right?

We ate boxes of Entenmann's cakes and Snack Wells cookies without guilt. Since there was no fat, they were not going to make us fat. At least that is what we were told.

Since I have struggled with my fair share of food issues and weight struggles, on my quest for skinny, I jacked up my metabolism really badly. When I finally heard the truth, I was determined to shift gears.

Rebuilding my metabolism by eating lots of delicious fatty foods and working out with heavy weights has been a journey—a journey you are about to go on yourself. Breaking bad habits isn't easy, but it is worth it.

This book is not about a "diet," it is a lifestyle program, to literally help you turn back the hands of time and age stronger, feel younger, look sexier, be happier, and heal your body.

Our bodies are all different. Our issues with food are not the same. What we need to do is mend our relationships with ourselves, our bodies, and our food. We need to love ourselves to health.

Lastly, this is not about body shaming, at all, this is about aging in health. But truthfully, the extra weight on your body is just not healthy. It is hard on your heart and joints, and is a precursor to many diseases. I want to give you hope, that you can change the path you are on. You can do a complete 180 and age stronger.

Draw the line in the sand and decide this is it! You deserve to be happy and confident, have more energy, and love your life!

This is not a sprint; it's a marathon and the finish line will be so worth your effort. Enjoy the journey.

FRIGHTENING FACTS!

Despite spending the most per capita on health care, the US is the least healthy country of the industrialized nations.

In 1980, the US ranked 11th in longevity, today we are about 43rd. Life expectancy has been lowered for the third year in a row, this is the first downward trend in about twenty-five years. This means that children born today are not expected to live as long as their parents did. With all the medical advancements, this should be in reverse.

Many experts agree that degenerative disease is highly preventable. The American Cancer Society says that only five to ten percent of cancers are caused by genetics. One of every two men and one of every three women will receive a cancer diagnosis in their lifetime. [1]

The New York Times, summarizing The Framingham study results, stated, "that a large portion of people who suffer heart attacks have relatively low LDL cholesterol." [2] Yet how many people are popping cholesterol lowering drugs that just so happen to have the potential side effect of death from heart attack. The irony!

And the saddest prediction is one third to one half of the children today are expected to get type-2 diabetes in their lifetime.

The US is so worried about health care reform, yet they are spending trillions of dollars to treat disease, rather than prevent it.

> The doctor of the future will give no medicine but will interest his patients in the care of the human frame, in diet, and in the cause and prevention of disease."
>
> ~Thomas Edison

THE CONSPIRACY

What do the medical schools, the pharmaceutical industry, insurance companies, the FDA, and big food have in common? They are in the profit business and a bunch of pricks. Since the tax payers are funding their madness, the health of our people is suffering.

We have been manipulated and fed lies from the pharmaceutical mafia, insurance companies, big food, the FDA and the government. I honestly feel that they all care more about money than the health of our people.

Follow me here.

<u>Medical Schools and Pharma:</u>

In the early twentieth century, Andrew Carnegie and John D. Rockefeller owned pharmaceutical companies. In order to boost sales, they provided massive funding, upwards of $100 million, to drug-based schools. This forced the holistic based schools to fold.

Fast forward two hundred years, and the forgotten history of how modern medicine evolved, many doctors don't understand what Hippocrates was trying to say back in 431 BC, "Let food be thy medicine, and medicine be thy food." Nope, they mostly studied medication and surgery.

Thanks to good old TV commercials and 6-page magazine ads, patients are surrounded with the latest and greatest medicines, promising to cure all their problems. From high cholesterol to erectile dysfunction from Alzheimer's to diabetes.

So, this explains why our unknowing doctors are prescribing so many meds: this is what they learned in medical school and what their patients want.

Instead of teaching people about disease prevention through lifestyle changes, most doctors are in the symptom management business. Plus, they just don't have the time to spend educating their patients. Many only allocate 15 minutes per visit.

Instead of letting food be our medicine, they are prescribing pharmaceuticals, and feeding us these poisons. Now, I am not blaming doctors here. I believe that they went to med school to help people, to make a difference. The curriculum just doesn't include nutrition or lifestyle practices, so many just don't understand it. Even my Dad's cancer doctor told him that it doesn't matter what he eats. So, he sits at chemo and eats candy and cookies.

This is a great way to stay in business, right? Feed the patients sugar, which feeds the cancer, give them chemo to kill it, and the cancer keeps coming back.

The cost of medical treatment is soaring and the payments to doctors declining. My personal doctor has switched to more cosmetic procedures, so she can make the money she was used to back in the day.

To make it worse, why do the pharmaceutical companies reward doctors with decadent vacations? Are they bribing them to prescribe their brand of medication? Oh wait, the sunshine act "stopped" the payola. Or did it?

Insurance Companies

My brother was on a pill for Hep-C that cost $1000 a day. And my friend's husband had heart surgery for a screaming good deal: only $700,000. Who pays for this outrageous stuff?

Not the insurance companies. Nope, they are in the profit business, remember? They pass this cost onto the insurance holders. Our healthy family was paying over $2000 a month for health insurance and none of the best doctors would even take it. They paid out so little, it simply wasn't worth the doctor's time.

Another problem with insurance companies is they are too selective on what they cover. Health insurance pays for medications but not supplements. They cover Western medical doctors but not Naturopaths or Integrative physicians. Supplements and Holistic practitioners should be covered as well. Why discriminate? Doesn't it cost less money to prevent disease then it does to treat it?

How about insurance starts covering gym memberships, massages, meditation practices, Naturopath visits, acupuncture, and anything that will help the whole person prevent disease, decrease stress and heal the body holistically without drugs?

Naturopath or Integrative Physician looks at the whole body and at the root cause of the symptoms; they treat the whole person.

Most people will not choose this route sadly, because they only want to go to traditional doctors and take medications that are covered under their health insurance. When it would be cheaper for both the government and the individuals to heal the root cause and look at nutrition and lifestyle choices.

Simply put, we let insurance companies indirectly determine our treatment plans. America does not have a health care industry, but a sick care industry. Trillions of dollars are spent each year on fighting disease, wouldn't it be less expensive to focus on prevention?

The FDA

This agency allows expensive drugs on the market before they have received long term testing. Thousands of people are killed every year from toxic side-effects. Plus, they say it is illegal to heal with supplements or other lifestyle changes.

Big Food

In the book, *Omnivore's Dilemma*, Michael Pollan explains how the problem with food started when the American farmer separated the crops from the livestock. The farm used to be sustainable, meaning the livestock ate the crops and then fertilized them. It was a perfect ecosystem. [2]

Once separated, we ended up with filthy feed lots and genetically modified mono crops. The cows are unhealthy because they are fed corn, which they are unable to digest properly. These poor creatures live in piles of their own crap. It is awful. When we took the kids to Disneyland, we drove down highway 5, in central California. We passed a humungous feed lot and I could swear that the dog farted, but he wasn't even in the car.

Worse than that, my mother in law lives about a mile away from a manure farm and you can smell the stench all the way down the road. The animals are given hormones to grow faster and antibiotics to kill the disease in their bodies. Then we eat their meat, and these delicious chemicals transfer to our bloodstream.

You are what you eat, and you are what your food eats.

Researchers can trace the glyphosate (Roundup) laden corn that a cow consumes to the human who ate the cow.

And sorry vegans, the problem is not just about the meat. Even the crops we consume contain pesticides, herbicides, and lack most vitamins, minerals, and phytonutrients that they used to have. In most cases, soil is only fertilized with three different minerals: nitrogen, phosphorus, and potassium. The produce is picked green, thrown in a truck and gassed while it is transported across the country. This way when it appears on your supermarket shelf, it is "ready to eat." Clearly, they are missing all those juicy nutrients that would develop had the produce had the chance to grow to maturity.

Even the amount of vitamin C in a modern-day orange, only contains about 10% of the vitamin C from that same orange 100 years ago.

The government is subsidizing the corn, wheat, and soy industries, in a huge way. In a typical supermarket, these 3 ingredients are found in 80% of the store. These inflammatory foods make us fat and sick.

So, instead of spending government money on producing organic, pasture-raised, healthy food, they are spending money on genetically-modified, processed crap.

And the food companies prey on the innocent. They produce TV commercials and print media in order persuade us to purchase their lab-designed frankenfoods. They make false claims that mislead the uninformed consumer.

When you read things like Heart Healthy, Whole Grains, No Trans Fat, All Natural, Low Sugar, Low Fat, Low Carb, approved by the American Heart Association, Gluten Free, Cholesterol Free, Fat Free, Real Fruit, it sounds healthy, right?

Worse yet, the advertisements prey on our children, so they are begging us to buy them all this crappy food too. The food dyes and sugar are really messing with our kids and affecting their performance at school and their behavior at home.

Processed food is making people sick. It is full of chemicals and genetically-modified ingredients and is stripped of nutrients. It creates inflammation in our bodies and fat on our thighs! So, what is the point of eating this garbage?

When you go to the grocery store, what is eighty percent of the food on the shelves? Processed crap! This is not food at all. Read a label and tell me if you can even pronounce most of those words, let alone know what they really are.

Our bodies do not know how to metabolize these chemicals, and I believe they are a huge cause of disease. Our cells need real vitamins, minerals, and antioxidants, to renew and divide. These chemicals and preservatives are toxic to that process and our bodies don't know what to do with them.

A local chiropractor has had a fast food hamburger on display in his office for several years now. Surprisingly, it has not grown mold. hmmm

On Howstuffworks.com I found this crazy list of the "Top 10 Groceries Americans Buy."[4] It is no wonder our country is so sick.

- Soda
- Cereal
- Frozen Dinners
- Salty Snacks (chips, pretzels, "cheese" puffs)
- Milk
- Laundry detergent

- Eggs
- Peanut butter and jelly
- Deli meat
- Bread

Most of the food on this list has sugar and preservatives and is highly processed. The bread will spike your blood sugar more than simply eating a spoon of table sugar! Let's take a closer look.

10. <u>Soda</u>—A typical can of soda contains thirty-three grams of sugar from high fructose corn syrup (HFCS for short) and phosphoric acid

HFCS is a manufactured sweetener and absorbed by the body much differently than cane sugar, which grows in the field. Simply put, the way your body digests this (food-like substance) causes insulin spikes (far greater than regular sugar) and a fatty liver.[5] All sugar is not created equally, and HFCS is the worst.

Phosphoric acid, used for rust removal, is highly acidic, can chew up your teeth and bones, and harms your kidneys.[6] Have you seen those viral YouTube videos showing people cleaning rust off their toilets or bumpers with Coke? Imagine what it does to your insides.

Diet Coke is not much better since it is sweetened with the toxic aspartame. Watch the documentary Food Matters to understand what I mean.

9. <u>Cereal</u>—The most popular cereal at my local grocery store is Honey Nut Cheerios, which has nine grams of sugar per three-quarter cup. Its recommended serving size seemed rather small, so I did an experiment. I poured the Cheerios into a typical cereal bowl, thinking that there would be two portions. And guess what? There were three. This means you are probably consuming closer to twenty-seven grams of sugar in a standard bowl of cereal.

Then you add milk, which adds another thirteen grams of sugar per cup. That is a lot of sugar in the morning. What a great way to set off your day and send the kiddos off to school. Frosted flakes are the #2 top seller with twelve grams of sugar per three-quarter cup.[7]

What other ingredients will you find in a box of "cholesterol-lowering" cheerios? Trisodium phosphate! Look that one up. I remember buying TSP to clean my bathroom. Maybe it cleans the cholesterol off your arteries the same way, or maybe not.

8. Frozen Dinners—When I went to the grocery store to research frozen meals, Healthy Choice was a name that stood out. I checked the label to find these ingredients: hydrolyzed corn, wheat gluten, and soy protein. There you have it! Corn, wheat and soy, the 3 most highly-funded crops the government subsidizes, and they are the highest GMO (genetically-modified) crops.

About 95% of the population has a gluten sensitivity and don't even know it. Gluten is hidden EVERYWHERE. If you consume a diet of whole foods, you will be safe from this inflammatory shit storm.

Several years ago, I took a stool test for gluten sensitivity. Not that I thought I was gluten sensitive, but if I was going to recommend my clients take the test, I needed to know how it worked. Yes, you have to poop in a bowl, freeze it, and then mail it. My kids were completely grossed out that I put poop in the freezer.

My results were surprising. Anything above 10 is gluten sensitive, I was 178! The lab recommended that I eat a permanent and strict gluten-free diet. Thankfully, this has been pretty easy, since 95% of my diet is whole foods.

7. Salty Snacks—Many people think pretzels are the healthiest option here. Well, they are wrong. First off, they contain gluten and carbs. Even if you eat carbs, they are not the healthy kind. Pretzels are high on the glycemic index, 83 to be exact. This is higher than any other salty snack I can find. So, noshing on these babies will help you grow that midsection quite rapidly.

The only salty snacks I recommend are nuts and pork rinds (a pasture-raised brand). When you add guacamole, the glycemic load of the entire snack decreases.

Don't worry, if you are thinking, "glycemic what?" We will talk about glycemic index and load in the next chapter.

6. <u>Milk</u> –I don't drink or recommend this highly acidic beverage, which is intended for baby cows.

Osteoporosis risk increases with milk consumption, believe it or not. Stay with me on this one. Milk is acidic. Our bodies are very smart and will try to neutralize this acidity. When you get heartburn, you take Tums, which has the active ingredient of calcium. Where is the body going to find stored calcium to neutralize the acidity in the milk? Your bones!

The states with the highest incidence of osteoporosis happen to be the biggest milk drinkers. Imagine that!

"According to a new study in the journal BMJ, the research found that consuming more milk was linked to greater risk of bone fractures and to earlier mortality."[8]

4. <u>Eggs</u> – Finally, a grocery I like. Pastured eggs are amazing and the reason why I have backyard chickens. I even endured the hell of cleaning up chicken poop all over my back patio for several years, until my hubby finally built a fence to contain them.

My girls lay the most amazing eggs. The yolks are a deep gold and deliciously creamy. Once in a while, I get an egg with a double yolk, which I call a keto egg.

Eggs are the least expensive complete source of protein and they taste great. The labeling may be confusing with terms thrown around like organic, cage free, all-natural, and pastured. Just make sure you purchase the best kind you can afford.

3. <u>Peanut Butter</u> – This is also on my "good foods" list. However, the commercial brands of peanut butter, which are full of sugar and hydrogenated oils, are not. Why do the food manufacturers add these crappy ingredients to the jar? My feeling is that the higher the sugar content, the more addictive the substance.

Look for brands that just contain peanuts and salt. I prefer organic here as peanuts are a high pesticide crop. Caution – peanut butter may contain traces of mold. If you have a sensitivity, be cautious.

2. Deli Meat – Full of nitrates and nitrites, which are not great. Cook real chicken or turkey, slice it up, and eat this instead.

1. Bread – The glycemic index of "whole wheat bread" is 71, not much lower than wonder bread, which is 73. The crazy thing is Coca Cola scores a 63; so essentially, eating a piece of bread will spike your blood sugar faster than drinking a coke. But isn't "whole wheat" bread supposed to be healthy?[9]

Essentially what is happening here is that people are filling up on macronutrients (calories), which feed their belly, but very few micronutrients (vitamins and minerals), which feed their body at a cellular level.

Since our bodies are made up of cells and we need micronutrients to create healthy ones, we are starving our bodies and never satisfied. Many people are overfed and undernourished. Over a million cells renew and divide every hour, and they need these micronutrients to be healthy. If micronutrients are not present, shit happens, both inflammation and free radical damage. Wherever your body has its weak point, symptoms will show up.

"Research has linked growing waistlines to a number of different sources, including processed foods, sodas and high-carbohydrate diets. Risks associated with belly fat in aging adults includes an elevated risk of cardiovascular disease and cancer.

Researchers have actually predicted obesity will overtake smoking as a leading cause of cancer deaths, and recent statistics suggest we're well on our way to seeing that prediction come true as obesity among our youth is triggering a steep rise in obesity-related cancers at ever-younger ages." [10]

~Dr. Joseph Mercola

JUST LIKE CRACK

And you are addicted to it! This may sound harsh, but I tell you the truth: sugar is a highly addictive substance and is making America the unhealthiest country on the planet.

Think about it: how many times have you had just one cookie or one piece of licorice? It's like crack—we just can't stop at one bite!

High-sugar foods stimulate the brain just like drugs do. In a study, laboratory "rats find Oreos just as addictive as cocaine because the cookies stimulate the brain in the same way some drugs do. The rats went first for the cream in the middle, just like lots of human Oreo consumers."[11]

The Oreos activated more neurons in the brain pleasure centers than cocaine or morphine. No wonder people can't eat just one; they love that high and feeling of euphoria.

Our brain is looking for pleasure. Sugary foods create that pleasure by releasing tryptophan, which is the precursor to serotonin, the feel-good hormone. So, when we get stressed out and are seeking that feel-good serotonin, to calm us down, we reach for a bag of cookies or a pint of Ben & Jerry's.

An adult woman should only consume six teaspoons a day of sugar. If you drink a can of soda, you have already doubled your allotment. Check this out:

- Sprite = 13 ½ tsp
- Vitamin Water = 8 tsp
- Ice Cream = 7 tsp
- Blueberry Muffin = 7 tsp
- Doughnut = 3 tsp

Do you truly understand what happens when you eat sugar-laden food or drinks? And did you realize that many non-sugar, carby foods do this exact same thing?

Here is the life of a typical American:

Breakfast: Cereal, OJ, and toast (or Starbucks mocha and muffin.) After eating this high glycemic meal, your blood sugar spikes and the body declares an emergency because of too much sugar. The pancreas secretes insulin to lower your blood sugar, but oftentimes this insulin response gets the blood sugar too low.

Snack: By 10am you are hungry again. You get weak and shaky because you need some more sugar. This is why they invented vending machines, which is filled with more crap. Things like cookies and candy, chips and pretzels (which may as well be sugar because they have the same effect on your blood). So, you grab your fix and go about the rest of your morning.

Lunch: Out comes the sandwich, chips, and fruit. It spikes your blood sugar again. If you look at a chart with your blood sugar levels, it looks like a big zigzag. Eating sugar leads to craving more sugar, and it's like a big sugar roller coaster.

As a child or teenager, you can handle these spikes; however, as we age, our bodies become immune to our own insulin and the excess gets stored as fat. Have you noticed your waist thickening as you age? This is excess insulin and known as insulin resistance or Syndrome X.

The solution is keeping your blood sugar stable, in a nice even range, not too high and not too low. This will help minimize the "crack", I mean sugar cravings.

Most of you girls know that sugar is not good for you. But I bet you don't even realize how much sugar is in so-called healthy foods. All carbohydrates metabolize into glucose.

One trick is understanding the Glycemic Index. This is a great way to judge whether a food affects your blood sugar or not.

Glucose is the benchmark at 100 on the GI index. And at the other end of the spectrum is olive oil with a low GI of 0. The lower the glycemic index the less effect it has on your blood sugar and the less insulin is released. For example:

<u>High Glycemic Foods:</u> Baked goods, white bread, potatoes, bagels, white rice, many cereals.

<u>Moderate Glycemic Foods</u>: Brown rice, banana, sucrose, apricots, whole-wheat pasta, popcorn.

<u>Low Glycemic Foods:</u> Meat, eggs, butter, oil, fibrous veggies, seeds, butter, cheese, Greek yogurt, & nuts.

When you consume low glycemic food, your blood sugar stays stable, and insulin release is minimized. Insulin is your fat storage hormone and all the excess insulin is stored around your waist. By ditching the high and moderate glycemic foods, your muffin top will begin to disappear.

The opposite of insulin is glucagon; this is the fat releasing hormone and it works opposite insulin. As the insulin levels drop, glucagon goes up and you will begin to release your fluffy belly and flabby butt.

One way to test your daily level of hunger out for yourself is a breakfast experiment. One day have a healthy breakfast (my favorite is eggs with bacon, spinach and avocado). Then record how you feel right after you eat, and how long until you are hungry again, and how you feel between meals that day.

Then, on another day, have a typical American breakfast of a muffin, cereal, and orange juice. Record how you feel afterwards, pay attention to when you are hungry again.

Did you notice a different response on each of these days? Which do you prefer?

Sugar also creates inflammation in your body. This is the root of all disease and is a precursor to type-2 diabetes. The inflammation remains in your body for up to three days after you spike your blood sugar.

Sugar also leads to:

- Type-2 Diabetes
- Heart Disease

- Kidney Disease
- Cancer
- Obesity
- Liver disease
- Irritability
- Lack of focus
- Energy crashes[12]

So, before putting that bite of sugar or carbs into your mouth, think about how short the pleasure that comes from eating the treat will really last... and weigh it against the long-term effects. Is it worth it?

CHALLENGE: Clean out the kitchen and throw out all sugary, carby, inflammatory foods.

> "Sugar is eight times as addictive as cocaine. And what's interesting is that while cocaine and heroin activate only one spot for pleasure in the brain, sugar lights up the brain like a pinball machine."[13]
>
> ~Dr. Mark Hyman

You Stuff Your Feelings!

And eat when you aren't hungry!

I remember in freshman year, when my boyfriend and I broke up. My heart was broken, and my favorite spoon couldn't keep itself out of the cookie dough. I didn't even bother to bake the cookies to ease the heartbreak. I just ate the dough out of my mom's Pyrex batter bowl.

Think about this. What do you do when you are:

- Cold? Bundle up.
- Thirsty? Drink water.
- Have to pee? Run to the bathroom.
- Tired? Go to sleep.
- Depressed? Eat.
- Stressed? Eat.
- Bored? Eat.
- Lonely? Eat.

Notice a pattern here? So often we use food for stuffing away feelings instead of really feeling them. This is a real problem.

For example, something happens at work, which stresses you out, you go home and pig out mindlessly on whatever you can get your hands on. Maybe it's a pint of ice cream, bag of cookies, or a pizza.

But then you wake up the next morning with the dreaded regret hangover. "Why did I eat that whole carton of ice cream? Why did I sit on the couch and binge watch Netflix all night and eat that whole bag of chips?

The problem is still there. Whatever happened to create those miserable feelings is now worse. Feel the feelings; don't try and stuff them away!

It is normal to have uncomfortable feelings: sadness, stress, disappointment, unhappiness, anger, and frustration. It's part of life. When you try to stuff them away, they do not magically disappear into that carton of ice cream.

Be mindful and feel your feelings, journal about them, process the emotions, and work on the solution. So often we focus all our energy on the problem and attract more problems. Instead of focusing on the problem, brainstorm the solution. What you think about, you bring about.

Take back your power! Don't let people or situations derail you from creating true health.

CHALLENGE: Other than hunger, list all the reasons you eat. Now list what can you do instead to work your way through that feeling. For example, when you are bored, take a walk or call a friend.

"Feelings are actual sensations that we can literally feel in out body. For example, when you are experiencing anger, you might feel tightnessin your jaw. They are like signals that, when interpreted correctly, can point you to your next steps.

Feeling your feelings is actually really simple and the worst thing that will happen is the feeling itself. Your feelings will not hurt you, but avoiding them does. "[14]

~Christie Inge

STRESSVILLE SUCKS

And you aren't coping well.

Living in Silicon Valley is pretty hectic. So many of us are commuting in horrible traffic and working 50+ hours a week. The big corporate campuses are even building dental clinics onsite so that you don't have to leave work to get your teeth cleaned.

Many women are caring for children and elderly parents, fighting health issues, dealing with financial stress, having marriage problems, or just lacking the energy to create a fulfilled life. It's bananas!

Everyone is so dang stressed out and too busy to do anything about it. I say that we live in Busyland and it has nothing to do with putting on Mickey Mouse ears and having a fun day at Disneyland.

It sucks when you run into someone you haven't seen in a while and say, "Hey, how are you doing?" And they say, "Oh man, I have just been so busy." I think that is just the rudest answer. It's as if to say, "I've got no time for you."

Stress kills! We all have stress in one way or another, and we must learn how to manage it. What exactly does stress do to your body? Web Cleveland Clinic posted: "Stress that continues without relief can lead to a condition called distress—a negative stress reaction. Distress can lead to physical symptoms including headaches, upset stomach, elevated blood pressure, chest pain, and problems sleeping. Research suggests that stress also can bring on or worsen certain symptoms or diseases." [15]

Plus, stress makes you fat! When you get stressed out, your body releases a hormone called cortisol; which has been linked to fat storage. So, the more you let stress wreak havoc in your life, the more fat will store around your middle.

"Stress can play a part in problems such as headaches, high blood pressure, heart problems, diabetes, skin conditions, asthma, arthritis, depression, and anxiety." [16]

With all of these scary side effects of stress, you would think we would all be mantra-chanting yogis.

How do you deal with the stress in your life? Do you use food to cope with this feeling, or do you deal with it in a more effective way?

One of my favorite ways to deal with stress is to exercise. One time, when I was tapering for a race and my trainer told me to rest and not doing any exercise, my kids were begging me to go to the gym. I guess I was a little cranky! Even going for a walk will soothe the nerves.

Some great stress busters are meditation, yoga, massage, and breathing practices. You can really calm your nerves by simply taking a few deep breaths in through your nose and out through your nose.

CHALLENGE: Create a plan that you can practice in order to calm the stressors in your life.

> "FOOD is the most widely abused anti-anxiety drug in America, and EXERCISE is the most potent, yet underutilized antidepressant." [17]
> ~Bill Phillips

FAKE, PHONY, PHOTOSHOP

When I was a young girl, I had Farrah Fawcett's swimsuit poster hanging on the back of my bedroom door. Seems a bit odd, looking back. In my mind, she was the epitome of a beautiful woman. She was thin, had gorgeous teeth and amazing hair.

Fast forward 20 years later, my husband can't wait to see the Sports Illustrated Swim Suit Edition. When we were first married, this made me feel a little inferior to these stunning women.

What do you consider to be the modern "ideal" woman? Open up any magazine and what do you see? Thin women, stunning hair and makeup, dressed in gorgeous clothes, perfect skin, and no wrinkles. So many women strive to look like this ideal. But is it really possible?

Do you know how many of these pictures are created? In the modeling industry and the quest for thin, many women simply do not eat. While some are naturally slim, many will starve themselves to get that desired look. Others have the funds to hire a personal trainer and chef to prepare their healthy meals and make them sweat off the rest.

To make things worse, we have Photoshop and airbrushing. I have seen where they take an average pretty girl, and with makeup and Photoshop they transform her into a ravishing beauty. They even lengthened her neck and widened her eyes.

It makes me crazy how distorted our perceptions are. We focus on what is abnormal or unnatural instead of what is real. It is really almost a slap in the face to the model, having to use photoshop to make her face appealing. Won't a little makeup be enough.

Then we look at the "ideal" body. Many of these models are what we call skinny fat. Meaning they are thin yet, have no muscles. An old friend of mine, that worked in the modeling industry in New York, said these girls are under a lot of pressure and it's just not healthy.

Since "strong is the new skinny", I sincerely hope we are changing the trend and will start seeing more fit and natural looking models in our media soon.

Another pet peeve of mine is aging and plastic surgery. Why can't we just age gracefully and embrace our laugh lines and forehead wrinkles?

Years ago, plastic surgery was used primarily by movie stars, but now it is easily available to middle class women as well. There are numerous things for anti-aging such as Botox, Juvederm, and collagen. You can make your nose smaller, your chin more prominent, your boobs bigger, smaller or perkier, get butt implants, cheek bone implants, liposuction, tummy tucks, or fuller lips.

Oftentimes people get plastic surgery and no longer resemble themselves. Or they get those silly, puffy lips and look like a duck. One day, I ran into a woman at TJ Maxx who called my name. I smiled and said hello, but I did not recognize her at all. Thank God she started talking about her son, and I put two and two together and realized who she was. She had so much "work" done on her face that she no longer resembled herself.

Even though I hate my thin lips and my big nose, I refuse to distort my face like that. And would be scared to death that if I decided to fix them and died on the operating table. What would my kids say? "Mom died because she was so vain and wanted to make her nose smaller."

The pressure to conform to the media's ideal woman is too much for many girls and women to compete with.

What can we do to end this cycle? I say change expectations and focus on fit and healthy. Go for strong instead of skinny. Embrace your fine lines and decide to love yourself where you are.

"Living as a perfectionist means thinking and living in "black and white" – there are no grey areas. You are either perfect with your diet, or you throw in the towel and completely screw it up, all while shaming yourself. Perfectionism is the death of happiness. It's impossible to feel happy and at peace with yourself when you are on a constant path of self-sabotage." [18]

~Samantha Skelly

You Love Making Excuses

Excuses are like armpits. Everyone has two of them and they both stink.

I had so many excuses when I was going through my tough years. I was unloved, I would start on Monday, I was too busy, blah blah blah.

When I start working with a new client and they give up because "life got busy", I feel so bad for them. They let "stuff" get in their way. Sometimes I have to say, do you want me to just listen to you vent and enable you? Or do you want me to call you out and coach you to success?

When you make excuses, the only person you are hurting is YOURSELF! You can create results or excuses, but you can't have both.

Who is watching you on your journey? Do you want them to see you fail? Be a good example of true health to your children, spouse, and friends. Would you want them to give up on themselves and their goals? My guess is you wouldn't. So why do you give up on yours?

The only way to truly fail is to quit! Decide that failure is not an option. Decide that what you want to achieve is more important than your excuses.

People are quitters by nature. Think about this. Most gym memberships go unused and the gym owners count on that. They sell way more memberships then the capacity of their gym, allowing for a large flake ratio. Do not be in this statistic and flake out on what you truly want to achieve.

So today, draw the line in the sand, step over it, and leave all your excuses on the other side!

Seriously, you can make an excuse, or you can make a commitment. You will never have the results you desire when excuses stand in your way. Keep your goal at the top of your mind every single day.

Below are some common excuses I hear:

<u>"I can't afford to eat healthy"</u>

Such a common phrase! I do understand why people think this way, when you can drive through McDonalds and purchase a value meal for $3 it may seem like quite the deal.

Or when you go into the grocery store and see a box of hamburger helper for $2.49 and buy some ground beef for $2.49 a pound, you can feed a few people for $5.

With these two examples, what are you really feeding your body? Just a bunch of empty calories, devoid of micronutrients, loaded with carbs, sugar and chemicals.

However, if you purchase a whole chicken and some broccoli, you can make a balanced meal and you will be eating whole foods, high in vitamins and minerals, and high in fiber (to help you poop and clean out your system). You might be spending a teeny bit more, but you are feeding your body a whole lot more...this is the TRUE Value Meal

The reason that processed and fast foods are so inexpensive is because most of their ingredients are made from soy, wheat, and corn. These crops are subsidized by the government, making them very cheap to grow and they are genetically modified; which is not good in my humble opinion.

When you eat processed foods, they are usually higher in carbs and you are hungry a few hours later. Now you have to eat again which will cost you more money. In the whole foods example, you will stay fuller longer.

You are going to either pay now or pay later. Either pay for healthy, clean foods now, or pay the doctor later. Live a vibrant, high-energy life now, or live a sick, dragging ass life later. Pay the farmer now or pay pharma later.

<u>"I have to cook for my kids and husband."</u>

Why is this an excuse? If you really love your kids and husband, stop feeding them crap. If you shouldn't be eating it, then why would you let them eat it?

Trust me, I fed my kids junk food all the time. I used to tease my sister in law, when she would pack my nephews would chicken, brown rice and green beans instead of peanut butter and jelly. Turns out that she was the smarter one after-all.

Help your family create good habits asap because bad ones are so hard to break.

<u>"I'm too busy"</u>

So, prep your food on Sunday...it will end up saving you time and money. Take the time now and save time later.

Imagine never having to throw rotten vegetables or expired condiments away. Imagine going to the grocery store and only buying the things on your list for the week.

We all have the same 24 hours in a day. By organizing your time, and planning your life, you will be happier at the end of the week. When you are healthy, you have more energy and free time to enjoy the things you love.

CHALLENGE –List the excuses you are making to not incorporate the healthy habits you need to reach your goals? What benefits would you experience if you did incorporate these healthy habits into your life?

BALANCE IS NOT BS

Many people think that achieving true health is all about eating less and exercising more. However, it is not that simple.

Do you ever feel like you are on a hamster wheel? Like you wake up, go to work, come home, cook dinner, and go to bed. Only to repeat the same things the next day. It's kind of like the movie ground hog day.

And on the weekend, we do yard work, clean house, cook, and deal with typical family drama. We oftentimes don't nourish ourselves and take special time-out to feed our souls.

We spend too much time taking care of everyone else's needs and neglect our own. This creates an imbalance and leaves us feeling. We often pour our energies into things that don't light us up and make us feel good.

The answer to this issue is feeding your body with primary food.

Have you heard this term before? When I ask people in my seminars what this is, they always say things like vegetables, fruit, meat, and grains.

Joshua Rosenthal, founder of my nutrition school, The Institute for Integrative Nutrition states, "Primary Food is more than what is on your plate. It is healthy relationships, regular physical activity, a fulfilling career and a spiritual practice can fill your soul and satisfy your hunger for life."[19]

There are many aspects of our lives that make us feel complete, feed our soul, bring us joy, and make us more fulfilled. Oftentimes when one of those areas is broken, we turn to food to "fix" the problem.

You know what I mean right? What is the first thing you did after your last breakup? Did it involve my two friends, Ben and Jerry?

Noticing and acknowledging areas in our lives that need improvement is the first step to creating more happiness. We will talk about the solution for this later in the book. For now, just notice your sticky points.

Take a look at the list below. Read all of the different categories and reflect on your own life, evaluating each area. Now rate them on a scale of 1–10 based on your level of happiness in each of these categories. Rate a 10 for awesome, a 5 for pretty good, and a 1 for awful.

1. Career
2. Home Life
3. Relationships
4. Finances
5. Fitness
6. Sleep
7. Passion and Purpose
8. General Health
9. Food

When you look at your honest scores, how does it make you feel? Which areas would you like to improve? Most likely, there are things in your life that could use some help, and that is why you are reading this book. The goal is to help you get to a higher level of happiness.

Morning routines are a very helpful way to create balance in your life. Starting your day off with loving self-care and clearing your head, will give you peace throughout the day. With practice, you can make it so automatic you don't even think about it, like brushing your teeth. Well, at least I hope you brush your teeth. By adding in new habits and practicing them every day, they become a ritual and will help you create results.

CHALLENGE: Choose two areas on this list that you would like to focus on first. Write down three ideas that you can implement to start improving each of them.

> "If you are not getting the primary food you need, eating all the food in the world won't satisfy your hunger." [20]
> ~ Joshua Rosenthal

PART 2

GET OFF THE NAIL

There is a story of a man who had a dog that howled all day and all night.
A stranger asked the man, "Why is your dog howling all the time?
The man replied, "He is sitting on a nail."
So, the stranger asked, "Well why doesn't he get off of it?"
The man replied, "Guess it doesn't hurt bad enough."

TAKE BACK YOUR POWER

When I was on Weight Watchers, I would not eat or drink before the meeting or I would skip it if I had gained weight. The number on the scale would determine if I would even attend the meeting. Too high? Go back to bed. Just right? Wear the lightest clothes possible and be the first one to weigh in so I could drink my coffee.

Then I worked with this popular Personal Trainer. He had this crazy weight loss challenge where he wrote everyone's name on this big white board and wat they weight every week. Needless to say, I sat that one out. When he kept pushing me, I just didn't come back.

A year later, I taught a weight loss workshop, I didn't make the participants weigh in weekly. It was optional (because I wanted them to keep coming back and learn the lessons being taught).

I was what I called "scale sensitive." The number on the scale would determine my mood for the day. If it was a low number, I did the happy dance. If it was high, I was down in the dumps all day.

One day, a friend posted this quote on Facebook and I died laughing. This became the entire motivation for writing this book. I always hated the scale and planned on writing this book about throwing it away.

> **Why weigh yourself when you could just set yourself on fire then roll in broken glass and feel the same way?**

However, my eyes were opened when I was doing research and found that most people who are successful with keeping their weight off, weighed in daily![21] I was so surprised! Then I realized that since they were enjoying success, they must know a secret. They didn't get all emotional and whiny over the number on the scale. Nope, they owned their power!

They looked at the number on the scale as SIMPLY INFORMATION!

- A way to tweak the path they were on.
- A way to gauge if what they were eating was working, or not!
- A way to figure out how much their suitcase weighs so they don't pay a premium on Delta.

Just like a pilot who is flying from San Francisco to New York City. Do you think it's a straight line? No fricken way! The winds and pressure are frequently taking the plane off course and the pilot must adjust the airplane accordingly. Just as we must adjust our eating and movement practices based on the results we are achieving.

After reading these studies, I was like, BINGO. I realized I had been doing it all wrong and decided to change. Reclaim my power, be honest about my food, and eat to live not live to eat. Be mindful about my hunger, my emotions and my food choices. I choose to fill my body with all the good stuff so I can crowd out the crap!

I don't even eat much lettuce in my salads anymore. Why take up the stomach real estate with water and fiber? I rather eat nutrient dense veggies as my salad base and save the lettuce for my rabbit.

Remind yourself that the numbers on the scale are only short term, because you are loving yourself to health. And the scale only tells part of the story. You are not what you weigh.

Keep in mind that if your joy is completely tied to your weight, your journey is going to be tough. Make things simple by avoiding negative mindsets about your body and place your attention on the positive work you are doing to enhance your health and to age stronger.

Transformation is not linear, and the mirror is not reality. So how about taking a photo of yourself in a bathing suit or underwear in the same spot every week?

Sometimes when we start exercising and building muscle on our bodies, the number on the scale doesn't change and we get bummed out. However, a tape measure and photo can show inches lost and proves that you are one step closer to fitting into those sexy jeans!

Would you rather lose an inch or a pound? What do you think weighs more? A pound of muscle or a pound of fat? That was a trick question!

So many people think muscle weighs more than fat. Well I am here to tell you that a pound of muscle and a pound of fat weigh the exact same: a pound. The muscle just takes up a lot less space in your jeans, which translates to a smaller size. Plus, it fills them out in the right places.

You must own your power. Let the scale be a tool and nothing more. Don't let anything have power over you: no people, no food, and no feelings. Be like Dr. Spock and control your emotions or they will control you.

CONTROL YOUR THOUGHTS

My husband used to be a news junkie. He woke up to KCBS news radio every morning and listened to it all day when he was driving around for his business. He was always stressed out.

Until one night, he heard an infomercial about Tony Robbins and spent money we didn't have to buy his *Personal Power* course.

After just a few days, he felt amazing. Not only was he not putting that stressful crap into his mind, he was replacing it with encouraging words. These cassettes literally changed his life.

Everything we do and every word we speak starts with a thought. You must control these thoughts. Our subconscious mind believes everything you feed it. So, we must feed it the things we want more of in our life.

What we see with our eyes and hear with our ears influences our thoughts. What we choose to watch on TV, listen to on the radio, or look at in a magazine may determine our actions.

We must choose to feed our minds the things that nourish and support us. Instead of reading a gossip magazine, read a health & fitness magazine where you will get good ideas for recipes or workouts. Instead of listening to the news on the radio, listen to a personal growth CD.

How many times have you thought negative thoughts about your body or about your life in general? Have you heard about the law of attraction? Or have you read the book *The Secret*?

The premise behind the law of attraction is that what we focus on, we attract into our lives. When we focus on what we want in our life, we will attract more of it. So often we worry about things and focus on negative thoughts, so we attract more negative outcomes. That is why some call it the snowball effect.

Nothing in life is static. We are either growing or we are dying. Grabbing fast food, then sitting in front of the TV for hours, numbing out the stress from the day is dying.

Filling our mind learning wonderful new ideas in the car on the way home from work and then going to the gym is growing.

Which will you choose?

CHALLENGE: Write down the negative thoughts you have. Next create a positive thought to replace it. Create a pattern interrupt and the next time one of these negative thoughts comes into your head, replace it with the positive one.

> "Whether you think you can, or thixnk you can't, you are right." [22]
>
> ~Henry Ford

Focus on Strong, Not Skinny

The new popular saying is "Strong is the new Skinny." Honestly, do we really need a new skinny? I think strong is way the hell better than skinny!

My two best friends growing up were very skinny. I tried for years and years to be like them, to be skinny, and just never made it. The constant struggle to reach that goal really messed me up. I had no self-worth or happiness, always striving for a different size and never being satisfied.

I ran and did high-impact aerobics, so much that I got terrible shin splints. That didn't even stop me. I would dose up on Advil and workout anyways. The physical therapist was my new best friend. I alternated between running and injuries, over and over throughout many years, filling up his bank account while I was at it.

One day, 20 years later, I woke the heck up! Instead of beating up my body with pounding the pavement, I went on a reinvention tour, like Janet Jackson, and decided to change my focus from running to weights. From thin to strong. The only running I did was a little bit in boot camp, and that was mostly sprints.

I realized that not only do we women need a strong body, but we also need a strong mind. I believe that by creating a strong body, a strong mind will follow.

We must love ourselves for who we are and not let anyone or anything ruin our mojo and determine how we feel about ourselves.

Many of us let stressful circumstances control the way we feel. We turn to unhealthy habits to cope with difficult feelings like stress, boredom, anger, and sadness. These feelings make the pint of Ben & Jerry's call your name!

Think about it, why do we let people take away our power, control our emotions, or ruin our mojo? When we do, we let them win! We need to put ourselves back into the driver's seat of our lives. Take back our personal power.

When my kids got their black belts, they had to read the *Book of Zen* and write meaningful quotes. One of the most popular was a Chinese Proverb "Control your emotions, or they will control you." [23]

Decide now to put your big girl pants on, and instead of letting toxic people, the scale, or any other outside influences take away your power, be strong.

I bet you are thinking, "if only it was that easy!" Trust me, I can sympathize with you on that. It's not easy, because we have been reacting to our circumstances for most of our lives, and old habits die hard. We must learn to respond to our circumstances with compassion for ourselves.

When you give someone else your power, by letting him or her control your emotions, you are reacting instead of responding. Next time, be mindful, take a deep breath, process the situation, and respond with grace instead. Think before you speak; the pause is good. Often this calmness will get their goat because they are trying to get a reaction out of you!

Just put on your Wonder Woman bracelets and block their crap.

All my life I let people affect the way I felt about myself. I was searching for acceptance and thought, if only I was skinny. So, I kept searching for that magic number on the scale. When I was much older, I finally realized that number didn't mean anything. That number was not going to define me. As long as I was "healthy," I was OK.

Now don't get me wrong, this is not an excuse to be overweight, I want you to be healthy. Healthy and Strong!

PUT YOUR OXYGEN MASK ON FIRST

As a busy mom, I have frequently sacrificed my needs and desires for my family. It's very natural that we want our kids to have the very best. But we don't have to let ourselves go in the meantime.

If you really want to love yourself to health, you need to learn how to *truly* love yourself and that starts with self-care. If you are like many women, you are thinking, what the heck is self-care? Well, I am here to tell ya!

Imagine that you bring a brand-new baby home from the hospital. What do you do with her? Snuggle her like crazy, kiss her all over, give her warm baths, and then rock her to sleep.

All those loving moments, right? Think about how you feel loving up that little baby girl. Warm and fuzzy and truly happy. That is what you need to do for yourself as well. When you practice nourishing self-care, you are showing love to yourself. And that inner child, craves this love so badly. Give it to her daily.

The world needs you and the gifts you have to offer. You are unique; there is nobody like you and please know that *you are beautifully and wonderfully made.*

To prove this to yourself, do this mirror exercise. Look in the mirror for several minutes. Starting with your eyes, the window of your soul. Send loving thoughts to that inner child who dwells deep within. Notice the pattern on your iris, the colors, and the whites of your eyes, are they bright and clear? Next, shift your gaze to your eyelashes, and eyelids. Next notice your forehead and your wrinkles and your hair

Look at your nose, your cheeks, your lips, your teeth, smile at yourself, frown. Which do you like better? Look at your teeth, your ears. Do you know why God gave us two ears and one mouth? So that we listen more than we talk.

Listen to your breath, to your inner voice. What are you telling yourself? Love yourself and how you were uniquely created, as nobody looks just like you.

Did you know that your eyes are a window to your soul? When I practiced Bikram yoga, we were instructed to stare into our own eyes for the first 30 minutes of class and listen to our breath. Not an easy thing to do.

Each time you shift your gaze to another body part, take a deep breath in through your nose. Breathe in love, joy, peace, compassion, and confidence. Then exhale through your mouth judgement, stress, frustration, and insignificance.

Now step back and look at your body with love. It is your temple; the only true home you will live in for all your days on the earth. See your neck that holds up that heavy head, that wonderful creative, analytical mind. Look at your shoulders and arms that give great hugs.

Stare at your hands that are so important to all of your daily tasks. Look at your chest, which holds your heart. See your tummy. This is the place where our lives began. Look at your legs that support you on your journey through life. Look at your feet, which hold you up as you walk through the days.

You have probably lived in at least two different houses in your life. But your body is the only home you will ever have. Are you supporting it?

When something happens to your house, like a toilet gets plugged or the heater stops working, do you repair it? Sometimes we even have to call in a professional to make the repairs for us.

Are you caring for your body like you do your house and making the necessary repairs? Are you feeding it healthy food, exercising, and drinking lots of water? Choose to love yourself the same way you would love that precious baby.

CHALLENGE: Do the mirror exercise and record your thoughts in your journal. Plan a self-care outing for this week.

Sticktoitiveness

In order to achieve success in life, we must have a plan. Set one up for all aspects of your life: food, fitness, sleep, and self-care. Promise yourself that you will stick to your plan as an important priority for yourself. Be committed to what you really want to achieve.

Every weekend, look ahead and plan your meals and grocery list based on what foods you will eat in the coming week. This will not only save you money, it will also save you time.

The grocery store can often be our worst enemy. But if we know how to shop with a list, it can be our best friend. Take a look at the special foods in the back of the book, and make sure to include them in most of your meals.

Either first thing in the morning, or the night before, plan out exactly what you are going to eat that day. If you have a busy day, maybe you should pack up your meals and snacks the night before.

The main reason most people don't exercise is because they are "too busy". So, if you also plan your weekly exercise schedule, as if it is an important appointment with yourself, then it will already have an allotted time. This is an important part in self-care. Instead of meeting a friend for lunch, how about meeting for an exercise class or a walk? This will be something you can look forward to.

Make bedtime part of a plan too - not just going to sleep when you feel tired. Schedule your sleep for at least 7-9 hours a night. And if that is just virtually impossible, then at least supplement with a nap! Catnaps, walks, and meditation will boost your energy for the rest of the day.

Make self-care a priority! Plan at least one little treat each day. Maybe a pedicure, a foot rub, reading a juicy novel, watch a fun movie, or a soak in the tub! Light candles and make your time special and pampering!

DO IT: Make your plan for the coming week: food, fitness, sleep, and self-care.

MAKE FITNESS FUN

Remember, you are not a number.... you are a beautiful human being with bones, muscles, organs, and maybe some extra fluff, waiting to be used for energy! Burned off while you enjoy moving your body!

One of the best strategies for sticking to a program is having a buddy participating alongside of you. This way you can meet up for workouts, share recipes, encourage each other, celebrate your successes together, and have fun on your day off.

Or you can create a contest at work. Many companies have fitness challenges or weight loss challenges. Make it fun! You can throw money in the pot and whoever has the highest percentage of body fat shed wins the money!

When I go to the gym at 5:30 am, there are tons of people walking on the treadmill, riding the elliptical, and spinning on the bikes. What do you think their goal is? Heart health? Fat burning? Stress reduction?

No matter what your goal, moving your body is an important part of this plan. Heart disease is the number one killer in the world, your heart is a muscle that loves exercise.

Many thin people don't exercise and that is not good. They think they look fine, so why bother?

Here's what I mean...I was hiking up a steep 2-mile hill with a skinny friend. I was blazing up the hill and my friend was huffing and puffing, feeling dizzy and needed to stop and rest often. Which one do you want to be?

Here's what exercise does for your body:

- Gives you energy and makes you more alert
- Creates an endorphin rush
- Makes you relaxed
- Decreases depression

- Suppresses sugar cravings
- Cleans your lymph system due to increased deep breathing
- Sweating increases the lymphatic flow which cleans out more toxins
- Improves your immune system
- Reduces the risk of diabetes, heart disease & cancer
- Lowers blood pressure and blood fats
- Increases your metabolism

So, if you lack motivation to workout, take some time to think of all these amazing benefits your body will receive when you do.

I suggest doing an experiment with different forms of exercise to find which you enjoy most. Join the gym and try out a variety of classes.

Once you find modes of exercise that you like, schedule it on your calendar. Make an appointment with yourself to get your groove on. First thing in the morning is my favorite time to exercise, that way the day doesn't get in the way and I have no excuse not to work out!

Once you establish a routine, it's going to be much easier. This requires you to be consistent. Have fun, be social, meet new friends, workout with a buddy. Find a way to enjoy moving your body!

Most weeks I am committed to working my ass off at Boot Camp 3 days, heavy weights 2 days, yoga 3 days, plus walking my dogs most evenings. I have this scheduled into my calendar.

If I cancel my workout, I am only hurting myself. Who are you hurting if you cancel yours?

Exercise releases endorphins (feel good hormones) and that is why it is essential to creating lasting lifestyle changes.

Walking is a great form of exercise. It is free and you can do it anywhere. It doesn't require fancy equipment or a gym membership. It is good for the heart and helps create strong bones. However, most people don't walk because they don't have anybody to go with, they aren't motivated, or maybe they can't get their butts off the couch.

Dr. Michael Roizen from the Cleveland Clinic says in his book, <u>You, The Owner's Manual,</u> that we should walk every day for 30 minutes rain or shine. [24]

Dogs and walking go hand in hand, because dogs love to walk, and they need us to take them! When my lab Ringo doesn't get his daily exercise, he is way too hyper and drives me nuts. However, when I take him and Rocky out for their walk, they are much more relaxed! Walking dogs is even a career for some people. So, if you don't have a dog of your own, you can volunteer to walk a friend's.

If you want a pet of your own, you can always go down to the local shelter and pick up a sweet pooch! Man's (and Woman's) best friend!!!

CHALLENGE: Take time right now to schedule your workouts for the coming week; write them in your calendar. If you have a buddy, have them write it down as well. If they cancel on you, do not let this be your excuse to cancel as well. Be like Nike and "Just Do It"!

"I'd rather be standing at the top of the hill that I just dominated unable to breathe, ready to puke, hair matted to my forehead, than at the bottom wondering what it would feel like."

~Unknown

Combat Temptation

My mother in law is the best ever! Sophie is a lovely lady who always means well. However, she is the worst when it comes to temptations. She is an absolutely incredible baker and loves to surprise my boys with treats. But what really happens when those sweet treats come though my front door? Tracee used to eat them, that's what! Store bought stuff is easy to resist, but Sophie's baking? OMG

There are a couple tricks I have learned in the past 30 years that have saved me from changing pant sizes. And the best one is out of sight, out of mind. I hide the treats in my lower oven or throw them away.

Another habit that gets people into trouble is tasting while cooking. Sometimes by the time you sit down at the dinner table, you are full, from picking at the food while cooking. In order to stop this behavior dead in its tracks, either brush your teeth or always have gum on hand, especially the minty kind. While chewing gum, your mouth is occupied, and the minty flavor will ruin the taste of anything you may be tempted to pop into your mouth.

One of my weaknesses is wine; I live on a Wine Trail for crying out loud. There is a winery in front of me, and behind me, grapes on all sides and I just LOVE relaxing with a glass of wine. So now, I fill my wine glass with sparkling water in between glasses...and it makes the pleasure last much longer.

You are a unique individual and therefore what tempts you will be different than what tempts others. Ask yourself these questions:

- What time of day am I most tempted?
- What events or circumstances cause me to be tempted?
- Who is with me when I am most tempted?
- How am I usually feeling when temptation strikes?

Becoming aware of the thoughts and feelings that lead to temptation will allow you to let go of them and replace them with empowering thoughts and feelings that drive you toward your goal. Make a game plan in advance! Mindfulness is a key to success in all things.

CHALLENGE: Take a few minutes right now and write down an answer for each of these questions. Next, create your empowering solution so you can respond in health the next time.

Opportunity may ring only once, but temptation leans on the doorbell.

Eat to Live, Don't Live to Eat

When I was pregnant, my husband had a growing business, and it was growing almost as fast as his waistline. He was a basket of nerves. He started eating fast food, donuts, pastries, chips, and candy. He would fantasize about what places he would drive through, what trees he would park under, and what donuts were hot out of the oven and at what time. HE LIVED TO EAT.

He was like a sneaky little kid hiding candy from his mommy. And he was so happy, until.... We went to Disneyland and he started people watching and noticed how many people were obese. They were dragging their bodies through the hot park and looked like they felt awful. Pete knew that was where he was headed. So, when we got home, he decided he wanted to change his lifestyle for good.

When we got back from that vacation, he started eating healthy food. No more fast food or donuts. He started eating whole food meals, taking vitamins, drinking smoothies, and exercising. At first it was hard. He could only do the elliptical machine for ten minutes and thought he was going to faint.

So now, 16 years later, my man is fit and trim, mountain biking many times a week and training for his 5th degree black belt. He now eats when hungry, listens to his body, and still allows for the occasional cheat meals.

Why must we eat? Simply put, the nutrients in food are the building blocks for our cells. All of our cells need energy to multiply and dive in health. Healthy foods create healthy cells and a healthy body.

Food choice is important here. Not all foods are created equal. Some will heal you and others will hurt you. We are bio-individuals, meaning our bodies may respond differently to different ways of eating.

People are not gaining weight by eating too much healthy food. It's more like too much sugar, processed food, chemicals, or fast food.

Create lasting lifestyle changes...a new you that will carry you through the rest of your life. Feed your muscles and feed your cells; just don't feed your waistline.

Next time you want to pig-out, ask yourself if you are REALLY hungry or if something else is going on? Drink a huge glass of water, wait 5 minutes and rate your hunger level again. Ask yourself what do you really need? Slow down, listen and be mindful with your decision.

> **What You Eat In Private,
> You Wear In Public.**
>
> ....
>
> **The Best Ab Exercise is 5 Sets
> of STOP Eating
> So Much Junk.**

MAKE A COMMITMENT

When we are on a "DIET" we are living in compliance. Thinking it's a temporary thing and you can't wait to be on the other side of it, for it to be over. You are either on the wagon or off the wagon; either on program or off. Diets are a temporary solution to a life-long problem

Conversely, when we change our lifestyle, we are making a permanent commitment to a healthier future. There is no wagon to fall off of because you are in control of the choices you make with each meal. There are no "rules" to follow, simply choices to make.

Compliance vs Commitment looks like this:

If you go on a typical diet, you usually feel deprived and want to chew your arm off. You cannot wait until it is over because you are not happy and white knuckling it through the whole processing. You are following the rules because someone told you they will work.

If you slip up before you reach your goals, you probably totally give up on why you started in the first place. This is compliance.

Conversely, when you truly understand what crappy foods, chemicals, and a sedentary lifestyle does for your body and are aware of the permanent damage you are creating, then you will commit to eating to heal your body.

Look to your right and left. Chances are you will see all kinds of people who are overweight, on medication and eating McDonalds.

I had a hard time giving up Diet Coke. I usually had one a day and enjoyed it. However, when I learned how bad it was for my body, I chose to get rid of it completely. This was a commitment. I wasn't giving it up because somebody told me to, but because I chose to.

You deserve to age in health, so commit to creating healthy habits and long-term lifestyle changes. You didn't get to your current status overnight, so it won't change overnight either.

EAT FAT AND FAST

Fat is not the enemy, sugar is.

When I was little, my parents were on the Atkins Diet and I was in heaven. I LOVED the salads with cheese and salami. Loved eating sardines with my dad, while he cheated with some Coors Lite. This was a fond memory indeed.

So, you can imagine my delight, three and a half years ago, when everything that I thought was true about nutrition was turned upside down. That Weight Watchers mentality that was so ingrained in my head shifted to the back to the old Atkins Diet principles, or so I thought.

While doing research for a nutritional protocol to help my mom with Hashimoto's and Alzheimer's diseases, I stumbled upon the ketogenic diet. At first, I was really quick to discard the notion that I could lose weight eating fat. Didn't fat make you fat? I was raised in the non-fat era, where carbs were praised, and fat was scorned.

We ate potatoes without butter, bagels without cream cheese, fat free cheese, mayo and boneless, skinless, tasteless chicken. Veggies were steamed and salads had fat free dressing.

Yet Americans were still sick and fat. I could not believe what I was reading, but the fat-free movement was clearly not working, so I was intrigued.

I dug in and did a ton of research. I listened to very scientific minds talk about the health benefits of this way of eating. Finally, after about 6 months of research, I tried it myself, and felt really good.

So, I decided to take my focus off of the scale and onto the healing of my body. Eating the high fat, keto way, was healing to my brain and body dysmorphia. I was so inspired to continue my healing journey. Now, it hasn't been perfect, please know this, but it has been so much better.

After hearing the wide array of health benefits people were experiencing, I decided to launch a podcast called Be Well, Be Keto: Ordinary People, Extraordinary Results. I am fortunate enough to interview so many amazing people who healed their body from various diseases by adopting a keto lifestyle. They are my inspiration.

I spoke with people who healed from depression to blood pressure issues. From bipolar disorder to hypothyroid. I interviewed doctors who helped their patients with cardiac health and cancer. And I interviewed athletes who are at the top of their game. All thanks to adopting the keto diet in addition to other lifestyle changes.

Please take a listen to the show to understand what I mean. It is called Be Well, Be Keto. Also, I have this cheat sheet I made and it's free for you in the book's bonus section.

The other component I am committed to is fasting, both intermittent and extended.

Fasting helps your body because your digestive system requires so much energy to perform its functions. And by giving the digestive system a rest, you are allowing that energy to be used elsewhere.

My favorite use of this energy is called autophagy. Dr. Axe says, "think of autophagy as a form of "self-eating," which might sound pretty scary but is actually your body's normal way of carrying out cellular renewal processes."

Intermittent Fasting, also called time restricted eating, is when you shorten your eating window to 6-8 hours. This means that you do not eat for 16-18 hours. By skipping breakfast and eating an early dinner, this is the simplest way to fast.

Another is one meal a day, or OMAD, where you eat in a one-hour window. This feels really good in my body and I do this frequently. I have so much energy during the day and then enjoy a nice dinner with a keto approved dessert.

Extended fasts are great for a deeper cleanse and intense autophagy. These are great to do in the spring, summer, and fall. However, your body does not love fasting in the winter. It wants to conserve energy when it is cold, so feed it warming foods.

I am committed to living a ketogenic lifestyle to keep my health as a priority and not have my genetics express. With my Dad having cancer for the 4th time, and mom losing her brain with Alzheimer's disease, I am fighting to age in health instead of disease. Combining this high-fat lifestyle with strength training, energy work and self-care practices, I intend to finish strong.

You can do it too. It is not too hard and it's never too late. If only my parents had stayed on the low carb Atkins, maybe they would not be fighting the diseases that they are today

My program, the High Energy Transformation, is a quick 21 day program follows the principles of this book And it will help you learn about transition your energy system to the keto diet, fasting, and movement. Check it out on the book bonus page.

"The advice to eat 6-8 times a day and to always eat breakfast even if you not hungry was never rooted in any science. There were no studies to show that this sort of advice actually worked. But if you don't eat, then people can't sell you products. So, eating all the time was good for business even if not good for your waistline." [25]

Dr. Jason Fung

FILL THE GAP

So, you now have the mindset and are ready to take your health to the highest level. You are making the commitment, right here, right now.

Good! There is No Fricken Way I'm going to let you back out now! You deserve this!

Now ask yourself, what is going on in your life that is making you turn to food to? What is the gap that you are filling with crap? It is time to crowd out? What foods, habits and people are not supporting your desired lifestyle? We all have things that would be better off disappearing. What are yours? Acknowledging them is your first step in healing.

When you fill your life with plenty of nourishing, healthy habits, you will heal your body and transform your metabolism. When you fill your tummy with healthy foods and your day with nourishing self-care, you will completely change the trajectory of your life.

So many people go on a deprivation, calorie restricted DIET and stick to it for the first week or month and lose weight. Then they fall off the wagon, give up on themselves, and go back to their old ways.

I have a secret, "THERE IS NO WAGON! We have cars now!"

Usually this is because they are looking at that diet as a short-term plan to get to their goals, they view it as a sacrifice, as suffering and they cannot wait for it to be over.

What I say is change your lifestyle, permanently. Those old habits were not serving you well. Eating carby, sugary, processed food is not good for your body, no matter how much you weigh. Starving yourself to a certain weight makes you hungry, grumpy, and it jacks up your metabolism. You need to feed your body and fix your broken metabolism.

My intention is to teach you how to fill your life and body up with so much good stuff there is simply no room for the garbage that is making you fat, sick, and unhappy.

Nourish your body with the foods and self-love that it is starving for and you will not want to dive into the late-night sugar binge.

Look at your body as a machine, as a well-loved and maintained Ferrari. Would you skimp out on the highest quality fuel, the loving rubdowns with the highest quality wax, and protecting it from the elements in a nice garage? Or would you let it get dirty, never change the oil, park it on the street, and let the elements rust it out?

Ok, maybe you are not into cars. So imagine you are an athlete. Would you eat potato chips and cookies while training, or ditch your workouts, skip the massages to rub out your muscles, or stay out all night partying? I doubt it.

You would feed your body high quality, energy producing foods, get lots of rest, and work out hard. You would love your body, so it will support you and love you right back.

During the Upcoming 21 days, you will learn how to do just that, simply and easily. Each day, you will learn a new healthy habit, a self-care practice, and about a new food. There are even recipes for you to enjoy. These practices and foods will help you to age stronger and feel younger.

PART 3

PREPARE

YOUR HEADSPACE

YOUR STORY

You need to examine where you have come from. How did you get to the place you are today? Why are you not where you want to be? This, my dear, is your story.

Before you embark on your health transformation, please write your story from as far back as you can remember until now. How did you get to this point? Did you hit rock bottom? This is for your eyes only, so spill the beans.

I know it seems corny and crazy, but trust me on this, it will help you move forward. It is a good ritual for releasing emotions.

After writing your entire story, read it. Feel the pain from your past and remember the past does not equal the future. You cannot change it, so acknowledge who you were as you prepare for who you are to become.

CHALLENGE: Get your journal and write your story in juicy detail. Go back as far as you can remember to dig deep into what loops in. your mind you have created. To recall the stories you have allowed yourself to believe.

DO NOT READ THE NEXT PAGE UNTIL YOU WRITE YOUR STORY. READY, SET, GO!

Your Vision

Congratulations on writing your story. Now if you are a rule breaker and didn't do it, please do not forget this important step. Stop reading and go write it now! Write it, and then read it out loud so you can feel the emotions come up.

How does it make you feel? Happy? Sad? Frustrated? Process those feelings and question them. Why are they lingering?

Assuming you read your letter, now you get to burn it, shred it, do whatever you want to get rid of that pain, that story you have lived with for all these years.

Everyone's story is different: some happy, some sad, some frustrating, and some painful. The good news is that it is your story and you can now create a new one!

But first, you need to decide what you want. Where are you going on your life's journey? Do you even know? Some people are so complacent and just accept where they are, that they have never even dreamed about where they would like to be.

Here is a famous story between the Cheshire Cat and Alice (from Wonderland):

Alice: Would you tell me, please, which way I ought to go from here?

The Cat: That depends a good deal on where you want to get to.

Alice: I don't much care where.

The Cat: Then it doesn't much matter which way you go.

So, in order for you to change, to create a better life, you must create your vision, you need to decide where you are going.

For this exercise, please find a quiet spot away from all distractions. Sit down with your eyes closed for 10 minutes or so and imagine your life. Imagine where you would like to be in a year from now. Try and see all the juicy details!

Have you heard the song Unwritten by Natasha Bedingfield? Every time I hear it, tears well up in my eyes and I get that lump in the back of my throat! Maybe play it in the background.

Somehow as adults we tend to stop dreaming as the stress of real life and responsibility gets in our way. Close your eyes and dream again! Put the pen to paper and write out what you want to see for yourself in a year from today.

What does your life look like? How do you feel? What can you do now that you couldn't do a year from now? How does your family respond? Has your energy improved? Are you enjoying improved intimacy with your spouse?

Write a journal entry with a date one year in the future. Act as if you are living that day and reflecting on how good your life is at this point. Be in the moment as if it was now. Don't leave out any juicy details. This will be for your eyes only.

GO DO IT NOW; YOUR FUTURE IS WAITING!

Print up this vision and keep it near your bed. Read it every morning when you wake up and every night before bed. Your subconscious mind doesn't know the difference between imagination and reality. So, when you fill it with this vision, your mind will find the way to create it.

When your days feel hard, and you want to give up, read it again and again. When you want to throw in the towel, you will be quitting on your dreams, and on your life that you deserve to live.

Remember, don't stress out about this homework! This is about LOVING Yourself to Health!

CHALLENGE: Get your journal and write your vision. Play the song Unwritten by Natasha Bedingfield so you can really get in the mood.

YOUR WHY

Most of the health industry is focused on the HOW TO! You know, you read the magazines: How to get bikini ready in 30 days, how to sculpt a 6-pack in 6 weeks, how to run a marathon in 2 months...blah blah blah.

Even though that is all very important, if it was enough, why is so much of America on medications, suffering with degenerative disease, in pain, exhausted, and overweight? "How To" simply does not work.

The solution is "WHY." A why that makes you cry!

WHY do you want to be healthy? WHY do you want to get fit? Why do you want more energy? WHY do you want to lose weight?

A WHY isn't a one size fits all. What matters most to one person is often different from another. We are all unique and need to find that deep, down core reason to draw the line in the sand, step over, and never look back!

What will inspire you to create true health, to heal your body, or to lose weight? Will your health reach the point where you have a disease such as diabetes or heart problems?

It is MUCH easier to prevent disease than it is to treat it.

Maybe you just want more energy, have the desire to be strong and fit for your children and spouse, be around for your grandchildren, or just look hot in a pair of jeans or on the beach.

Possibly you have always desired to be more fit, a smaller size, or you are simply sick and tired of being exhausted. Whatever encourages and motivates you, that is your anchor...that is your why!

Put your WHY in writing, on post it notes and stick them where you will see them throughout the day. Maybe post on the refrigerator, the pantry door, the bathroom mirror, your computer and in the car.

When you think you may want to give up and throw in the towel, read your why! Don't give up on yourself and your dreams! Remember you are loving yourself to health!

CHALLENGE: Write down WHY you must transform in your journal. Then write it on post its and tape to your bathroom mirror, your fridge, and your car dash...wherever you will see it often. This is your anchor!

"Imagine, if you will, being on your deathbed. And standing around your bed are the ghosts of the ideas, the dreams, the abilities, the talents given to you by life. And that you. for whatever reason, you never acted on those ideas, you never pursued that dream, you never used those talents, we never saw your leadership, you never used your voice, you never wrote that book. And there they are, standing around your bed looking at you with large, angry eyes, saying, "We came to you, and only you could have given us life! Now we must die with you forever." The question is: If you died today, what ideas, what dreams, what abilities, what talents, what gifts would die with you?" [26]

~Les Brown

DARE TO DREAM

Now that you know your Vision and your Why, it's time to build a picture of it: your Dream Board.

Maybe you have an old photo of you from a time when you were living your healthiest. Place that picture in a spot where you can look at it every day.

If you desire to hike a mountain, become a runner or have flat abs, find a picture that encourages you and post it up as inspiration. Where do you want to travel? What activities would you like to enjoy? Where do you want to live? What car do you want to drive? This is not just about health; this is about your dream life!

Discover what motivates you most so you can focus your subconscious mind on it frequently. Remember your subconscious doesn't know the difference between imagination and reality. Athletes visualize winning the race. Black belts visualize breaking the board. What will you visualize?

Have you ever constructed a dream board? This is such a fun project to do either alone or with some friends. Basically, you get a poster board and write a list of all the things you want to accomplish in your lifetime.

You can either search these images on the internet (Google images) or buy a bunch of magazines and cut out pictures.

So, build your dream board. What things do you want to do that you never thought possible? What vacations do you want to go on? How are you going to look on that favorite beach? What adventures do you enjoy? Hiking half dome, riding horses, cycling along the mountaintops, white water rafting?

As you start on your path to creating better health and shedding the extra weight, you will want to constantly stay committed to your why. Visualize your future life with your dream board and rekindle your passion every day.

CHALLENGE: Create your Dream Board, then post a picture in our Facebook Group: High Energy Girls

> "By representing your goals with pictures and images, you will actually strengthen and stimulate your emotions because your mind respons strongly to visual stimulation...and your emotions are the vibrational energy that activates the Law of Attraction. The saying "A picture is worth a thousand words," certainly holds true here." [27]
>
> ~Jack Canfield

PART 4

21 DAYS TO LOVE YOURSELF TO HEALTH

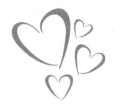

CROWD OUT THE CRAP

C – carbonated junk
R – refined sugars
A – artificial garbage
P – processed food-like substances

Remember when I say crowd out the crap, I mean fill yourself with so many good things, that there is NO ROOM for anything else!

How many days does it take to form a new habit? Most people say 21, so we will go with that. As you now understand, everything we do or don't do begins in our head, so we want to fill that baby up with some good old-fashioned LOVE!

Introducing 21 days of Crowding out the Crap. Love yourself and feed yourself and all the juicy details in between.

Try it on for size, see how it feels and always record your feelings in your journal. But commit to the practice so you can record the results and inspire others to change their life too!

At the end, you will print up a check list of all the tasty foods and self-care practices. Each week moving forward, make a game of how many foods and self-care things you can squeeze into your days. This will help you create permanent healthy habits.

CHALLENGE: What crap are you ready to crowd out? Write it in your journal AGAIN!

DAY 1 LOVE YOURSELF: BREATHING

Life or Death - we need our breath! Think about that for a minute. When we check a person to see if they are dead or alive, we notice if they are breathing.

Many people breathe short, shallow breaths. However, deep belly breathing has health benefits other than just delivering oxygen. Fortunately, we can train ourselves to switch over to this breathing style.

We do this breathing technique in Pilates and it's funny because we are trained to suck in our gut all the time, and in this type of breathing practice you fill your lungs and belly with oxygen, like a balloon and on the exhale, you contract your pelvic floor and blow out the air.

There are plenty of health benefits of practicing deep breathing. These include detoxifying, lymphatic drainage, releasing tension, improving blood, elevating moods, and weight control. [28]

A wonderful breathing exercise is to take 10 deep breaths before each meal. This will quiet down your busy day and allow you to be fully present to enjoy the nourishment you are giving your body.

This is one of the ways I work through a breathing exercise: Repeat 10 times.

- Inhale through your nose and count.
- Hold your breath for 2 times that count.
- Exhale slowly for 2 times that original count.

In yoga, my instructor has us engage in a different breathing practice. Simply cover your nostrils with your thumb and ring finger. You can rest your pointer and middle finger on your forehead.

Start off by taking a couple deep breaths through both nostrils and notice if one feels more open than the other. Next, inhale through your left nostril, while plugging your right nostril. Then cover your left nostril and exhale through your right. Then inhale through your right, and exhale through your left. Repeat this pattern about 10 times. Lastly, take a few deep breaths with both nostrils and notice if they are more balanced.

Either way you choose to practice deep breathing, it is a great practice to center yourself, calm your mind, and love yourself to health.

CHALLENGE: Take a 10-minute break and try both of these breathing practices right now. Record in your journal which you prefer and plan to practice one or both each day.

FEED YOURSELF: COFFEE

Coffee is one of my very favorite experiences. Not just for the energy boost to help me with my gym workouts, but the smell and taste are amazing.

The stimulant in coffee is caffeine and it can help people feel less tired and increase energy levels and the main reason why we need it for a morning kickstart.

There are many health benefits of coffee. The polyphenols and caffeine are beneficial in a variety of ways. Caffeine can boost the metabolic rate, therefore increasing fat burning in the body. Caffeine stimulates the nervous system, which breaks down your fat cells. Then they release into the blood as free fatty acids, and you can burn them as fuel.

According to Healthline.com: "the polyphenols found in coffee may help prevent a number of diseases, such as heart disease, cancer and type 2 diabetes ." [29]

Drinking coffee may protect you from Alzheimer's disease and dementia. There are studies that show that coffee drinkers have up to 65% lower risk in getting these diseases. With all these amazing health benefits, you can enjoy your cup of joe every morning.

My Keto Coffee

1 cup Organic Coffee
1 tsp MCT Oil
5 drops Stevia
Shake of Cinnamon

Place all ingredients into a glass blender and whip until frothy.

Iced Coffee Frappe

1 cup cold Organic Coffee
1 dropper of Stevia
1/2 cup Coconut Milk

Place all ingredients in blender and blend until ice is crushed completely.

"Coffee's effectiveness as a high-performance brain fuel makes it liquid gold, and it's not surprising that coffee's primary active ingredient, caffeine, is the globe's most commonly used psychoactice drug. The connection between caffeine's main botanical source – the coffee plant – and our own biochemistry is one of nature's best hacks." [30]

~Dave Asprey

Day 2 Love Yourself: Sleep

I love to sleep. Around 8:30, I head down the hall and get prepped to fall into my soft cozy bed. My hubby laughs at how attractive I look when I go to sleep. What with my mouth guard, ear plugs, eye mask and hair in a top knot, I look like a real babe!

But combine these with my magnesium pills and foot cream, I arm myself for an amazing night's sleep.

How do you sleep? Do you stay up late watching TV or try to get one more task on your to do list complete before you turn in? Does your alarm scream at you in the morning to wake up or do you wake up naturally, rested and ready to take on your day? How much sleep are you getting and how is this affecting your mood for the day?

Ideally, you want to be able to fall asleep quickly and sleep all night until your body wakes up naturally. Seven to nine hours is ideal for most. Sleeping during the hours of 11am to 3pm is key for rejuvenation.

If you are not getting the ideal amount of sleep, we need to figure out why. Sleep is critical for health. And lack of it is linked to increased risk of stroke, cancer, obesity, diabetes, brain deterioration, and bone loss.[31]

Melatonin is an important hormone and part of the sleep process. When the sun sets and it becomes dark, the brain starts producing melatonin, which prepares your body for rest and stimulates human growth hormone. But if light hits the eye, melatonin and HGH production shut down and the usual cellular repair that occurs while we sleep becomes disrupted.

In order to improve your sleep, start by making your room dark! Your alarm clock should have a red light, as this is the least stimulating color. Get as many electronics out of the room as possible, at least 6' away from your head! Charge your phone down the hall...far away from your bedroom. Unplug anything you do not need while you sleep. The electromagnetic frequencies these produce disrupt the delicate electrical system of the body. Turn off your wifi if possible.

Before falling asleep, do something peaceful and relaxing such as reading a book, deep breathing, light stretching, meditating, or prayer. Shut your mind off. Write in your journal before bed to mind dump and get all those thoughts on to paper so you don't need to be bothered with them while sleeping.

One of my favorite hacks is using this MagneZZZium sleep balm that my friend makes. Magnesium is known to be a muscle relaxer, and many people take the pills. But the balm absorbs into the blood stream quicker as it bypasses digestion. An Epsom salts bath works well too. The magnesium absorbs into the bloodstream via the skin.

Allow yourself the gift of a good night's sleep and see how much more productive you will be the next day!

We all live in Busyland and many people are sleep deprived. We are walking around like a bunch of Zombies (love Walking Dead) and this is sincerely hurting our bodies and hindering our performance during the day.

Sometimes people have a hard time turning off their mind and actually falling asleep. (I hear this is a sign of a High IQ) So the fact that I fall asleep easily isn't a good sign I imagine!

Here is a summary of my very favorite sleepy time tips:

- No electronics before bed
- Sleep in a VERY dark room
- Keep the temperature cool
- Play white noise
- Read a book with pages
- Have a relaxing bedtime routine
- Use a gratitude journal for happier dreams
- Keep a notepad by the bed in case a thought pops up
-

CHALLENGE: Create your bedtime routine. Start practicing it right away and notice how you feel.

"Many people gain weight in the summer. One main reason is because they skimp on sleep. It is easy to get 8-10 hours of sleep when it gets dark out at 4:30pm in January, but who wants to go to bed when it is light out? Not me!" [32]

~Maria Emmerich

FEED YOURSELF: BONE BROTH

Bone broth is all the rage these days because it has so many wonderful health benefits and is simple to make.

Unlike traditional chicken broth, chicken bone broth is thicker and gelatinous, especially when cold. It is made by slow cooking bones and allowing the marrow to be released into the broth. The marrow is a lovely, healing elixir that tastes delicious, and has many benefits.

One amazing benefit is that bone broth helps leaky gut syndrome. Scientists believe that the gelatin in the bones may seal up holes in the intestines.

Bone broth is a great source of glucosamine, which can help reduce, and treat joint pain. Chondroitin sulfate has been shown to potentially help with osteoarthritis. I even give it to my yellow lab, Rocky, who has arthritis in his back ankle. He does much better now that he takes this supplement.

Bone broth is a great source of collagen that may help tone your skin.

It also has glycine that can help you improve your sleep and ward off fatigue.

I love to cook once and eat three time. First, I roast a couple chickens for dinner. Then I remove all the meat from the carcasses and set aside to top my salad for the next day's lunch. Lastly, I use the carcass to make a healing bone broth.

Bone Broth Recipe

2 Chicken Carcasses
2 T Apple Cider Vinegar
Onion, sliced
1 T Garlic, chopped
2 stalks Celery, chopped
Rosemary Sprigs

Place all ingredients in crock pot and cover with water. Cook on low for 24-36 hours. The longer it cooks, the better. Strain and enjoy.

"Bone broth is known as a powerful food for promoting gut, skin, joint, and bone health. But to provide you these benefits, it should be made with bones and connective tissue from grass-fed, grass - finished beef bones or organic chicken bones, which contains beneficial protein, collagen, and amino acids." [33]

~Nick Mares: Kettle and Fire

Day 3 Love Yourself: Epsom Salt Bath

The Jacuzzi tub was invented for a reason! The water feels so good on my body that every time I take a warm bath, I fall asleep in it. I love lighting candles and hearing the splash of the water which soothes me right into lullaby land.

Since I exercise a lot, sometimes my muscles are achy, or my knees are sore and soaking in Epsom salts helps with this. I usually add 2 cups of these salts to my bath and soak for about 20 minutes.

The Epsom salts contain magnesium and sulfate. When you add them to your bath water, they simultaneously pull the salt and toxins from your body and replenish you with magnesium and sulfates.

The Epsom Salt Council lists these health benefits as well: [34]

Magnesium:

- Ease stress and improves sleep and concentration
- Help muscles and nerves function properly
- Regulate activity of 325+ enzymes
- Help prevent artery hardening and blood clots
- Make insulin more effective
- Reduce inflammation to relieve pain and muscle cramps
- Improve oxygen use

Sulfates:

- Flush toxins
- Improve absorption of nutrients
- Help form joint proteins, brain tissue and mucin proteins
- Help prevent or ease migraine headaches

Studies also show that since the heat of the bath warms your body, the "rapid decline in core body temperature increases the likelihood of sleep initiation." [35]

FEED YOURSELF: LEMON MILK

Even though our liver does a great job of detoxifying our body on its own, sometimes a little boost doesn't hurt.

Lemon milk is the perfect solution. Not only does it detox your liver, but the gallbladder too. And it tastes delicious.

Lemon milk does a great job and is known to help with the following:

- Detoxifies the liver
- Stimulates lymphatic drainage
- Contains anti-cancer and anti-tumor properties
- Boosts immunity
- Helps to decrease viral load and fight infection (lemon essential oil from the lemon rind is anti-viral)
- Improves absorption of nutrients
- Alleviates constipation and improves digestion (lemon juice helps to increase peristalsis which gets the bowels moving!)
- Healing leaky gut
- Improves energy
- May offer cardioprotective benefits (nutrients from the rind)
- May offer neuroprotective benefits (nutrients from the rind)
- Reduce or abolish swollen lymph nodes[36]

And it is super easy to make. When I first started drinking lemon milk, I would strain out the pulp This takes some time and since the pulp doesn't bother me, I choose to skip this step.

Lemon Milk

32 ounces Purified Water
2 T Extra Virgin Olive Oil
1 Organic Lemon, quartered
½ dropper Liquid Stevia

Place 16 ounces of water, oil, lemon, and stevia drops into a high-speed blender. Blend on high for about 2 minutes. Add remaining water blend until combined.

"Also, get back to a natural/seasonal rhythm—screen time is just as damaging to our mitochondria as is too much sugar or too many chemicals. Preferably, no screen time or light exposure after sunset outside of candlelight or use the groovy blue blocker glasses if you face that exposure. Get on a good sleep cycle—our body does its "clean up" between 11:00 pm and 3:00 am. If you are awake during that time, you are not taking out the garbage, and, therefore, adding more burden to your body. It's better to sleep at the front end of the night for five hours versus the latter end for eight. Example: 9:00 pm to 2:00 or 3:00 am does your body more-good than 2:00 to 10:00 am. You can see that immediately on blood glucose/ketone monitors and HRV devices if you don't believe me. Two nights of bad sleep or staying up past 11:00 pm increases insulin and insulin-like growth factor—which leads to obesity, endocrine disruption, Alzheimer's, and cancer to name a few." [37]

~Dr. Nasha Winters

Day 4 Love Yourself: Affirmations

Now that you really understand the power of your mind, how about we add some affirmations to your routine?

We have between 50,000 and 70,000 thoughts per day.[38] How many of your thoughts are positive happy thoughts? And how many are negative defeating thoughts?

The way you can get in the habit of thinking positive thoughts and feeding your mind some happy juju is by writing your list of affirmations and keeping them somewhere to read daily.

Here are some of mine:

- I have blessed many people in achieving true health
- I am a good listener, peaceful, and happy
- I am a financially prosperous woman
- I am healthy, lean, and strong
- I attract only healthy things into my life
- I am confident and bold, yet gentle and nurturing

CHALLENGE: Make a list of at least 3 affirmations, print the list and put it in a couple places where you can read it during your day!

Feed Yourself: Greens

Many people ask me why I have so much energy and I swear one of the reasons is because I have always been the salad queen. I have enjoyed chopped salads all my life and now I also add greens to my smoothies and soups.

Greens are high in vitamins K, A, and C – high in polyphenols. Bet you are wondering what the heck are polyphenols?

They protect the body's tissues against oxidative stress and associated pathologies such as cancers, coronary heart disease and inflammation.[39]

Raw greens are also full of enzymes, which help digest your food. When you eat foods high in enzymes, they lighten the typical work load of the digestion process and frees up your energy to be used elsewhere.

Rotating your greens is another important habit. The reason is each plant contains different nutrients and different micro toxins. By rotating, you are able to enjoy the unique nutritional profile of each green and not load up on any one particular toxin.

My favorite greens are

- Swiss Chard
- Spinach
- Red Leaf Lettuce
- Cilantro

Also try watercress, kale, romaine, green leaf lettuce, beet greens, collards, mustard greens, and parsley, arugula the list goes on!

Next time you are at the grocery store, purchase a new green or two that you haven't tried and then look up a yummy recipe to cook up that night.

The list below is called the Dirty Dozen and they are the highest pesticide crops. So be sure to buy organic as often as possible to avoid pesticide consumption.

Dirty Dozen

- Apples
- Strawberries
- Grapes
- Celery
- Peaches
- Spinach
- Sweet bell peppers

- Nectarines (imported)
- Cucumbers
- Cherry tomatoes
- Snap peas (imported)
- Potatoes

Foods on the Clean 15 are the lowest pesticides and you can go conventional, as they are relatively safe.

Clean 15

- Avocados
- Sweet corn
- Pineapples
- Cabbage
- Sweet peas (frozen)
- Onions
- Asparagus
- Mangoes
- Papayas
- Kiwi
- Eggplant
- Grapefruit
- Cantaloupe (domestic)
- Cauliflower
- Sweet potatoes[40]

Visit EWG's website to print up the list. http://www.ewg.org/foodnews/

Don't forget to bring it to the grocery store with you! When you do purchase any kind of produce, make sure you wash it very well. Your grocery store should have a proper veggie wash in the produce section.

Here are a couple of my favorite ways to eat my greens.

Green Smoothie

1-cup Water
½ cup Ice
1 serving Protein Powder
½ t Cinnamon
2 cups Greens

Blend until smooth

Sautéed Swiss Chard

1 bunch of Swiss Chard
1 chopped Onion
4 cloves Garlic
2 T Olive Oil
1 cup Chicken Bone Broth
Salt and Pepper to Taste

Sauté onion and garlic in olive oil using large pot. Fill pot with greens and bone broth. Cover and simmer 10-15 minutes.

And of course, there is always salad. **Lots of salad.**

DAY 5_LOVE YOURSELF: HYDRATE

Did you know that oftentimes, when you feel hungry, you are really simply thirsty? And if you are thirsty, you are already dehydrated. In American, 75% of people are chronically dehydrated.[41]

The health benefits of drinking water are almost too many to list. Since 60% of our body composition is water, it must be pretty important for bodily functions. Such as...

- Satisfies thirst
- Increases energy
- Boosts strength - muscles are full of water
- Improves joint health
- Flushes out toxins
- Plumps up skin, make you look less wrinkly
- Helps you poop
- Fills up your belly so you eat less
- Keeps your kidneys healthy
- Regulates body temperature

And the list goes on...so how much should we drink? Web MD says ".... we may not need 8 glasses...." [42]

What? That sounds like you could get away with less. And unless you only weigh 128 pounds I disagree. Eight glasses of 8 ounces is 64 ounces. Many fitness experts say a person should have ½ ounce per pound of body weight, minimum!

I like to drink a gallon or more of filtered water every day. How do I get it all in?

Well every morning, I brush my teeth and head down the hall for my delicious cup of coffee and while the coffee is brewing, I down 16 oz of lemon water with a tsp of salt.

Why lemon water? Well first off, it balances your PH, protects your immune system, flushes out toxins, aids digestion, reduces inflammation, aids in digestion, and more.[43]

If you add salt, you will give your body the electrolytes it will need on a keto diet. I use about a tsp of pink Himalayan sea salt in my lemon water every morning. And when I do not drink this, I feel the energy crash at the gym.

Next up, I fill my favorite one-liter stainless steel water bottle and put 4 hair ties around the top. Each time I refill the water bottle I take one off. So, by the end of the day, they are all gone, and that alone is a gallon.

If you drink one liter by 9, another by noon, one by 3, and the last by 6, then you will sleep well and not be up all night in the bathroom. Herbal teas such as hibiscus or green/mint count too.

Many factors increase your need for more water…. such as strenuous exercise, living in a hot climate, illness, drinking caffeinated beverages, or alcohol. The rule of thumb is to add 2 glasses for every serving of caffeine or alcohol.

What kind of water should we drink? Not those plastic bottles you get at the grocery store. You would be better off drinking from the hose.

There are many issues with those plastic water bottles. Like how long has that water been stored in the warehouse? Where did they procure the water in the first place? Is it just tap water? Was it exposed to extreme heat or cold where the plastic chemicals would be more apt to leach into the water?

The other thing to be careful of is fluoride and other chemicals in your water. Check the city water report to determine if your tap water is pure. We have a well, so have it tested regularly for toxins.

You also may consider getting a reverse osmosis. Aka RO, or a charcoal filter (such as a Brita). I LOVE my RO machine and it even produces alkaline water. It also pipes into my fridge, so my ice is clean too!

And please whatever you do, if you add one of those water flavorings packets, make sure it doesn't have aspartame! Go for the stevia drops instead.

My absolute favorite is bubble water. I have a soda stream and use it every single day as a wonderful treat. Enhanced water is amazing too. Simple add cucumbers, mint, lemon, orange, or strawberries to the water in the evening. Place it in the fridge overnight and wake up to flavorful water. It is a nice change or pace.

FEED YOURSELF: SALMON

Wild salmon is super healthy and high in Omega 3 fatty acids. Most of what you find in the stores is farm-raised, so choose wild Alaskan salmon when you can find it.

First off wild salmon is not only high in Omega 3's, it is a great source of vitamin B12, vitamin D, selenium, and B3. It is easier to digest than most protein sources, and it tastes great!

What is all the hype about Omega 3's? According to Web MD, "They may help lower the risk of heart disease, depression, dementia, and arthritis. Your body can't make them. You have to eat them or take supplements."[44]

One of the reasons I don't like to eat the farmed salmon is it grosses me out to think how they are raised: crowded, fed antibiotics, and dirty. The worst part is farmed salmon contain high levels of PCBs, polychlorinated biphenyls (PCBs), which according to PubMed are highly associated with cancer and other diseases.

It reminds me of that old Roseanne Roseannadanna skit from Saturday Night Live. When she says, "These fish are swimmin' in their own toilet."

I could be wrong but it pretty much grosses me out. At least the wild fish have a much larger toilet.

Mercury is a concern with salmon, since they are large fish. So, you may want to limit your intake to once a week.

Lastly, if you don't have a Traeger Grill, I highly recommend investing in one. They cook your food with wood pellets, so I feel it's much healthier than charcoal or propane. It is easy to turn on and makes the very best smoked salmon.

Smoked Salmon

1 large Salmon Filet
1/3 cup White Wine
1/3 cup Bragg's Liquid Aminos
1/3 cup Olive Oil
1T Paprika
1T Garlic Powder
½ T Cayenne

Marinate large, wild salmon filet for a couple hours. Place on smoker (or grill on extra low heat) skin side down, for 2-3 hours. Tastes great served over salad or eaten fresh off the grill.

Fish Taco Salad

1 large Salmon Filet
1Bag of Shredded Cabbage/coleslaw mix
½ cup Chipotle Mayo
¼ cup Apple Cider Vinegar
2 droppers Stevia
Salt and Pepper to taste
Avocado, sliced.

Spread salmon lightly with olive oil. Heat grill to medium heat and grill fish on each side for about 4 minutes or until opaque. Meanwhile, mix mayo, apple cider vinegar, and stevia together. Toss with cabbage and sprinkle with salt and pepper.

DAY 6 LOVE YOURSELF: GRATITUDE

My friend Shawn posted this on Facebook one day and it stopped me in my tracks. "What if you woke up today, and the only things left, were the things you were thankful for yesterday?" Wow – does that not shine a light on the importance of gratitude?

Or how about this? You have 2 children and give them each the same gift. The first one complained that it was the wrong color, too small, and not what he wanted. The other was full of kisses and hugs and said, "Thank you mommy, it is just what I wanted."

Which child will you be excited to give a gift to next time? I know which one I choose.

When we focus on the good things in life, we tend to see more good things. And there are always plenty of things to be grateful for. They say it is impossible to have gratitude and depression at the same time.

So, respond well my friend, find the good in your circumstances, and be grateful for all the little things. One of my favorite quotes is "A person's happiness or unhappiness does not depend on their situation, but on how they respond to it."

CHALLENGE: Every night, before you go to sleep, choose 3 things that you are thankful for from that day and record them in your journal. Reflect back often so you can remember how blessed you are.

FEED YOURSELF: GRASS-FED BEEF

You are what you eat, and you are what your food eats. The anatomy of a cow is designed so their proper food is grass. And that is what cows used to eat, prior to feed lots.

Grass fed cows eat chlorophyll containing grass and is higher in Omega 3 Fatty Acids. It is my very favorite source of protein.

Commercially raised cows are fed a diet of corn and grains to fatten them up. Researchers have found traces of herbicides, used to grow the corn and grain, in the blood of a human, after consuming factory beef. It certainly makes you think twice. My hubby prefers conventional steak, for the marbling and flavor. But, not me!

You really want to be careful because many products labeled grass fed, may be corn finished. If this is the case, you have no idea how long they were being fed grass and how long they were fed corn. When in doubt, always ask.

Please know this is not meant to create scare you. It is always better to eat any meat over processed foods.

Bulk Taco Seasoning

4 T Cumin
4 T Chile Powder
4 T Paprika
3 T Salt
3 T Granulated Onion
2 T Cayenne
1 T Garlic Powder
1 T Oregano

Mix well and store in jar. Brown a lb of ground beef. When half-way cooked, add 1 T of seasoning mix. Finish cooking until nice and crumbly.

Taco Salad

2 cups Lettuce, chopped
¼ cup Cilantro, chopped
4 ounces Taco Meat, cooked
1ounce Cheddar Cheese
½ Avocado
2 T Sour Cream
Hot Sauce to Taste

Combine all in bowl and mix well.

Day 7 Love Yourself: Meditate

In the mornings, after boot camp, I sit down to have coffee with God. This is my quiet time where I do my bible study, pray, then meditate.

No matter what your spiritual preference, it is so good for the soul to find a quiet time practice.

Some people think meditation is all granola, hippie, woo woo. And sadly, those people are missing out!

To simplify, meditation is just putting that busy little mind of yours on pause. It is quieting the voices in your head and helping you to be able to take that practice out into the real world so you can really live life in the present.

Meditation is a great stress coping mechanism and with practice, will bring other health benefits as well.

The easiest way is to use an app, like Calm or Mindspace. They both have free trial programs, so test each out and see which you prefer.

Zen Habits recommends, "Start with the Breath. Breathing deep slows the heart rate, relaxes the muscles, focuses the mind and is an ideal way to begin practice."[45]

Feel your body and the energy inside of you. Start with the toes, wiggle them and be thankful for the balance they bring to your daily movement. Next, flex your feet and reflect how they walk you through your life. Feel your legs, flex and then relax your muscles and notice how strong they are.

Repeat a similar process for the rest of your body. Be present and realize how awesome and powerful your body is. Notice how every part of your body depends on the other and how together each makes the other part better.

After you are fully relaxed, maybe focus on one intention that you want to be present in that day.

When your mind drifts off, notice it, and bring it back to your breath. Let the thought float away like a balloon in the sky!

When I teach fitness classes, at the very end of our cool down, we take a deep breath and then send out a blessing to someone. Darren Hardy calls (something like this) a mental love note. So how about finishing off your meditation with just that? Send a mental love note to someone who needs it. Afterwards, how about giving them a call?

FEED YOURSELF: BROCCOLI SPROUTS

Life begins in a seed. When you plant a broccoli seed, it grows into a beautiful broccoli plant in a few months. Alternatively, this same seed becomes an edible, nutrition filled sprout in just 5 days.

The nutritional content of this sprout is over 10 times more powerful than mature broccoli. So, it is easy to ingest more nutrition at one sitting when eating the sprouts.

According to the amazing blog of Dr. Josh Axe, Broccoli Sprouts:

1. May Fight and Prevent Cancer – including throat, lung, colon, prostate, breast, bladder, skin cancers
2. Might Benefit the Heart
3. Support Strong Bones
4. Might Help Fight H. pylori Infection
5. Detoxify the Body
6. May Improve Respiratory Function
7. Can Be Part of a Multiple Sclerosis Diet
8. Could Protect Your Brain[46]

To grow, simply purchase a seed sprouter at your local grocery store or online. Soak 1 T of broccoli seeds in water for about an hour. Spread in sprouter and cover with lid. Water every day. In about 3-5 days, you will have delicious sprouts. I prefer eating them when they are shorter and about 3 days old.

Ways to Enjoy:

Smoothie

1 cup Water
1 cup Coconut Milk
¼ cup Hemp Seeds
1 cup Organic Spinach
1 cup Broccoli Sprouts
½ cup Frozen Berries
1 Avocado
1 T Cocoa Powder
½ tsp Vanilla

Combine all ingredients into the base of a high-speed blender. Process on the "smoothie" mode or for at least 45 seconds on high until completely blended. The texture should be smooth and creamy.

Super Food Salad

1 cup Arugula
½ cup Watercress
½ cup Cilantro
¼ cup Broccoli Sprouts
½ Avocado
2 T Sprouted Pumpkin Seeds
2 T Avocado Oil Dressing

Chop all veggies and combine in bowl. Top with dressing and toss. Broccoli sprouts really absorb the dressing and add a nice texture.

DAY 8 LOVE YOURSELF: ENERGY WORK

Life force energy is important in many ancient cultures and is starting to gain popularity here. This energy is called Chi, Qi, or Prana.

At the very smallest point in the human body, is energy. The Chinese have been practicing energy medicine for about 5000 years and I am so surprised it's not used more in the US. I have been practicing Qi Gong and Tai Chi for several months. And I am a Reiki Level 2 Practitioner. Energy work is the future of medicine, as it is much easier to catch an issue at the earliest stages than it is to treat something fully manifested.

Every day, I practice a powerful form of Qi Gong called Pangu Shengong. According to the official website, "It was developed by Master Ou Wen Wei with a fundamental philosophy and practice rooted in kindness and benevolence. It is designed to absorb the beneficial energy of the sun and moon and the essence of the Qi of the universe, while regulating and intensifying life force and the immune system." [47]

This practice takes about 21 minutes a day and will cultivate energy into your body. I explain it by filling your energy bucket each day. Many things take energy out of our bucket, it is important to fill it up again to stay healthy.

Now this energy is different than the jumping up and down energy you may think of. This is the deep energy stored in all realms of our body, from emotional to spiritual, from etheric to mental. It is about your vibration you put out into the universe.

Reiki is another amazing way to work with energy. In many hospitals, they measure the energy of the patient, and if it's too low, they will perform Reiki on them to increase it. So many things can be released in your body with energy work. I love helping people clear energy blockages and increase their vibration with Reiki and Qi Gong.

FEED YOURSELF: EGGS

Living on a farm we raise our own chickens. They poop all over my yard, but the eggs are worth the extra effort to clean up after them. Eggs are the least expensive complete protein source you can buy. They are easy to cook and good for you!

There is a big controversy about the cholesterol content in the egg contributing to heart disease. Many experts say the cholesterol in the egg does not transfer to blood cholesterol. Our body needs cholesterol, and that is why the liver makes it for us. Cholesterol is the mother hormone. It produces pregnenolone which produces the sex hormones of progesterone, estrogen, testosterone, and DHEA. A big part of aging is a decrease in hormones. So why would anyone want to decrease cholesterol if they want to age younger.

Egg labeling is confusing and often deceptive. Types of eggs can be:

- Farm Fresh
- Cage Free
- Free-Range
- Organic
- Backyard Chickens

Farm fresh - means nothing to me since most chickens are raised on some sort of farm, duh. The humane society says chickens only need 67 square inches to live. Simply disgusting!

Cage Free – still live in the big factory farm, just not confined to a cage. They still may not see day light and are crowded and dirty.

Free Range- we are getting better. These hens are able to spend time outside. They love to forage for bugs and can live a more natural life.

Organic –both cage free and free range, no antibiotics unless the birds get sick.

Backyard chickens (pastured) – are the best. They live a humane lifestyle, foraging for bugs outside all day. And when the sun starts to set, they head for their coop. I feed mine vegetable scraps and use their poop to fertilize my garden.

Egg Cups

8 cups Power Greens, chopped
1 White Onion, chopped
12 Eggs
6 T Feta Cheese
1 Dash Cayenne, Onion Powder, Salt and Pepper

Heat Oven to 375. Spray muffin tin with olive oil.
Steam greens, drain, and chop. Divide evenly into muffin tins. Add 1/2 T chopped onion into each cup.

Mix eggs, whites, and season to taste. Pour egg mixture over veggies in muffin tin. Top with feta, dividing evenly.

Bake for 27-30 minutes. Let sit for 10 minutes and enjoy 3 whole cups for a serving. One egg cup has only 190 calories and 23 grams of protein.

Eggs Benedict

4 Eggs
1 ½ tsp Salt
1 tsp White Vinegar
4 cups Spinach
1 large Egg Yolk
2 tsp Lemon Juice
Pinch Cayenne Pepper
4 T Butter

Steam spinach until just wilted and drain. Boil water and add 1 tsp salt and 1 tsp vinegar. Lower heat to simmer. Using spoon, swirl water. Crack egg into center of swirl. Remove from heat and cover for 5 minutes. Lift egg out of water and serve over steamed spinach. Top with sauce.

Hollandaise Sauce: Blend egg yolk, lemon juice, cayenne, and salt in blender. While blender is running, pour in melted butter and blend until creamy. Add salt and pepper.

DAY 9 LOVE YOURSELF: CELLULAR NUTRITION

Simply put, every hour over a million new cells renew and divide. The difference between health and sickness is the quality of these cells.

The very oxygen that we breathe in everyday, that we need to fuel our organs, also causes damage to our cells. Think about what happens to an apple when you leave it on the counter. It turns brown, right? The air causes oxidation and discolors the apple and it gets mushy too.

That same thing happens inside our body every time we inhale. Oxidation comes from oxygen and free radicals occur. To combat those free radicals, and replace the missing electron, we need antioxidants.

We also need to boost our immune systems. The same immune system that fights those nasty bugs, like the flu and the common cold, fights off the cancer cells too.

When we decrease the inflammation in our body and boost our immune system, it's a win/win!

The solution is we MUST supplement. This does not mean you can drive through McDonalds and simply take your vitamins, and all will be good. Supplements are to SUPPLEMENT an already healthy diet.

Make sure that every day with your breakfast and with your dinner, you are taking high quality vitamins, minerals, omega 3's, vitamin D, and whatever else your body needs.

Please remember that all supplements are not created equal. You want something that is bioavailable and not a bedpan bullet (doesn't even get dissolved).

If we take care of our bodies, by eating lots of delicious nutritious foods, supplement with high quality supplements, and exercise, we nourish the cells of our body and create good health. And the need for medication will decrease.

CHALLENGE: Purchase some high-quality supplements and Omega 3 Fatty Acids.

Feed Yourself: Avocado

My favorite healthy fat has to be avocado. I love the creamy texture in my salads, omelets, or dipping chips into guacamole.

Avocados are loaded with vitamins and are considered very nutrient dense. Avocados are a source of monounsaturated fats, which can help lower bad LDL cholesterol and reduce risk for heart disease. [48]

Back in the low-fat days, I never ate avocado as I was brainwashed into thinking that they were fattening. Boy was I happy when I learned that fat does not make you fat!

Deviled Eggs
12 Eggs
1 Avocado
1 Lime
Cumin
Cayenne
Salt

Boil a dozen eggs until hard. Scoop out yolks and mash with an avocado. Sprinkle with cumin, cayenne, lime, and sea salt. Fill egg whites with yummy mixture.

Avocado Mousse

1 ripe Avocado
2 T Unsweetened Coconut Milk
1 T Cocoa Powder
6 Stevia Drops

Mix all in food processor, chill and enjoy. You can even freeze to make an "ice cream".

Guacamole

3 Avocados
¼ cup Onion, chopped
1 Jalapeno, chopped
¼ cup Cilantro, chopped
½ cup Cherry Tomatoes, quartered
1 Lime, juiced
½ tsp Sea Salt

Mash avocados and combine with remaining ingredients. Cover and chill.

> Never
>
> Give up on a dream
>
> Just because of the
>
> Time it will take to
>
> Accomplish It.
>
> The time will pass
>
> Anyway" [49]
>
> ~Earl Nightingale

Day 10 Love Yourself: Personal Growth

Nothing in life is stagnant. You are either growing or you are decaying. Which would you prefer?

The world is filled with news pollution. Everywhere we turn there is this shooting, that war, this recession, blah blah blah. There are also good things happening all around the world that we never get to hear about.

Instead of stressing out on all the bad things in the world that you can do nothing about, put your mind to work and grow your mind.

When I have to commute in Bay Area traffic, I enjoy the time to listen to podcasts or CD's to grow my knowledge and my mind. How many minutes or hours a day do you spend in your car? Instead of listening to news or mindless tunes, wouldn't it be better to listen to encouraging, thought provoking podcasts or CD's during that time?

Maybe when you return home from a long day at work, your attitude will be a little more joyful and you will be chillaxed around your family!

Instead of watching mind-numbing TV for hours on end, how about reading 10 pages of a fantastic book? Go to bed feeling uplifted and inspired instead of numb from media saturation. If you read 10 pages a night, that's 300 pages a month. You would be reading over 12 books in a year! Imagine if you even applied what you learned? You could create a whole new life for yourself.

There are so many wonderful authors out there who have written some amazing personal growth books and recorded incredible CD's. I love Darren Hardy, Tony Robbins, John Maxwell, Brendon Burchard, and Bob Proctor.... the list is endless.

Go to your local library and see what is available. I bet you will be pleasantly surprised.

CHALLENGE: Plan to Feed Your Mind Daily, 10 pages of reading, and 15 minutes of listening

FEED YOURSELF: BUTTER

Saturated fat was falsely demonized in the 60's when we were all told that saturated fat was linked to heart disease. So, we switched to margarine. We ate bread and potatoes, but no butter. Our veggies were steamed and tasteless. Yet heart disease remained the number one killer of both men and women. All the while our country got fatter and fatter.

New research indicates that saturated fat is indeed good for us and is important for hormone production. Even the USDA lifted their restrictions on saturated fat consumption in their latest guidelines.

Butyrate is the preferred fuel source for our large intestinal cells. This is especially important because it helps prevent and heal leaky gut syndrome. Intestinal permeability is considered by many the leading cause of inflammation in the body. This is most likely the rationale by how butyrate helps reduce auto-immunity and prevent cancer cell development. [50]

Grass-fed butter has much more Vitamin A than ordinary butter. Vitamin A is important because it nourishes our teeth, bones, and soft tissue, it also maintains our vision, mucus membranes and skin.

The fat found in butter is converted to energy for our body's muscles and organs. This process is more efficient than body fat being turned into ketones for fuel. The fat can also suppress our appetite, which can help when trying to lose weight.

Grass-fed butter is high in conjugated linoleic acid, which is a compound that can protect us from different types of cancer.

Don't fear the cholesterol, because we need it for healthy cellular function and to make key hormones. Cholesterol is vital for our brain and nervous system function.

If your body can tolerate dairy, butter is a great way to add flavor and healthy fats to your meals. My favorite brand is Kerrygold which is made from the milk of grass-fed cows in Ireland. I buy it at Costco or Trader Joe's.

Ways to Enjoy:

Mushroom Sauté

1 lb. Mushrooms, sliced
2 cloves garlic, minced
4 T Butter

Melt butter in pan. Sauté garlic until golden. Add sliced mushrooms and sauté. Serve over your favorite steak.

Butter Coffee

2 cups Coffee
1 tablespoon Grass Fed Unsalted Butter
1 tablespoon Organic Coconut Oil
1 dropper of Liquid Stevia
Shake of Cinnamon

Place all ingredients in blender and whip until frothy.

DAY 11 LOVE YOURSELF: STRETCHING/YOGA

Do you ever get out of the car and walk hunched over for a few minutes before being able to stand tall? Do you ever feel muscle tightness or soreness and don't have the range of motion you used to have?

Well no surprise. Most of the day we spend our time living in a little 2-foot box in front of us. Think about it. Our steering wheel, keyboard, stove top, and kitchen table are all 6-8 inches in front of us.

Most activities we enjoy during the day are in that little box and shortening our muscles. And those muscles are strong suckers. They have the ability to pull our bones out of socket and pull our tendons and ligaments out of whack.

We must stretch our bodies. Or risk aging as hunched over little old ladies. That is NOT what I have in mind. This is why I got certified to teach yoga.

Yoga is a fantastic practice because it not only stretches out your muscles and joints, it quiets your mind, focusing on your breath, and makes you in tune with the feelings in your body.

My favorite teachers practice Anusara Yoga and they always have a beautiful message to contemplate during the practice. Sending love to others, appreciating our bodies, and caring for our emotional and physical needs.

Ideally, I would love to practice yoga 3 times a week, and incorporate stretching every day.

My favorite stretch is to roll your shoulders back and down, clasp your hands near your butt, and pull hands up toward the ceiling. You can even bend forward if you like.

FEED YOURSELF: WALNUTS & ALMONDS

My husband grew up on 100 acres of walnut trees and so when we planted our orchard, he insisted we plant seven walnut trees. Even though I was never a big fan of walnuts while growing up, I have come to love these babies!

Walnuts are a fantastic source of Omega 3 fatty acids; this is why they look like little brains. They are also high in Copper and Manganese.

Most people use walnuts in baking, but I find them to be a great afternoon snack or on top of a salad.

These nuts are a snack I enjoy at least 3 times a week. They taste good, are convenient to keep in your purse for emergencies, and have lots of health benefits, including:

Almonds also have great health benefits.

- Lowers cholesterol
- Reduces Cancer Risk
- Reduces the risk for heart disease[51]

A one hundred calorie serving is about 19 almonds. In order to avoid eating more, pre-pack little containers with 19 almonds, and keep one in your purse and pantry for snack times.[52]

One word of caution, many of us can overeat nuts by not being mindful. One day, I went to Trader Joe's as I forgot my lunch. And next thing I knew, ¾ of the bag of macadamia nuts was gone. Lesson learned.

My new rule with nuts is I eat them only on a salad or yogurt. Never by the handful, unless they are proportioned and that is all I have.

One is too many and 100 never enough, applies for me with nuts. I must be mindful when eating them.

Way to Enjoy:

Oven Roasted Nuts

Place nuts oven safe pan and into cold oven. Heat oven to 300 and set timer to 10. When timer goes off, turn off oven and let nuts cool in oven.
Taste great on top of a salad or as a snack.

Greek Yogurt Parfait:

1 cup Unsweetened Greek Yogurt
1 T Vanilla Protein Powder
1 shake of Cinnamon
2 T Walnuts, chopped coarse
½ cup Berries

Combine yogurt with protein powder and cinnamon. Place in glass. Top with ½ cup berries and 2T chopped walnuts.

Almond Milk

Soak 1 cup of almonds in water overnight.

In the morning drain and rinse well. Place soaked nuts in a high-powered blender with 2 cups of water.

Blend on the highest speed. Add 2 more cups and blend again.

Strain the pulp and give it to your chickens. Place remaining liquid in refer.

DAY 12 LOVE YOURSELF: NATURE HIKE

Sometimes when our life seems to be falling down around us, focusing on the simple beauty of creation gives us joy. My favorite way to do this is go on a hike in the mountains.

I realize that not all of us live near the mountains or even have hills within driving distance. But nature exists every time we step outdoors. Look up at the beautiful blue sky, puffy white clouds, sunsets, sunrises, lightening, rain, the moon, and rainbows. Please don't look at the sun though; as this will hurt your eyes.

Look around at trees and wonder how old they are. I love big trees and wonder what story they would tell if they could. Don't forget the flowers! In my state, we have the California poppy and what I love about this gorgeous flower is how it closes up at night and opens wide during the day. It makes me appreciate how even plants need their rest time.

Animals and birds are another interesting part of nature. While you probably don't have wild animals in your area (unlike us who have boars, coyotes, and mountain lions) there are always birds! I love seeing them in formation flying "south for the winter."

Connect with nature regularly. It may be as wonderful as taking a hike, walking on the beach, or simply strolling in your neighborhood and smelling the flowers.

FEED YOURSELF: APPLE CIDER VINEGAR

ACV is a popular tonic in the kitchen of a health coach! It is antibacterial, antiviral, and antifungal. It will help with a sore throat, balance your digestive system, and even whiten your teeth.[53]

The reason I feel it is important to include a vinegar in my list of healthy foods is because I am the salad queen and recommend eating a big salad every day. Since it's the "healthiest" of all vinegars, I almost always use it in salad dressing recipes. Remember the Big Salad on the TV show: Seinfeld?

My new favorite way to drink ACV is add a tablespoon to a glass of sparkling water. It tastes a bit like kombucha (more on that later), which of course is an acquired taste.

My favorite brand is Braggs Organic Raw Apple Cider Vinegar. It looks a bit nasty, and you may think it's spoiled, but that cloud you see in the bottle is a live "mother" and it contains part of the health benefits.

Other benefits found on the Bragg Website:

- Rich in enzymes & potassium
- Supports a healthy immune system
- Helps control weight
- Promotes digestion & ph Balance
- Helps soothe dry throats
- Helps maintain healthy skin
- Helps promote youthful, healthy bodies
- Soothes irritated skin
- Relieves muscle pain from exercise [54]

Love Your Liver

2 quarts purified water
¼ cup Bragg's Apple Cider Vinegar
large knob of peeled ginger
1-2T stevia
1t Himalayan sea salt

Blend in blender, strain, and store in refrigerator. [55]

DAY 13 LOVE YOURSELF: MINDFULNESS

Have you ever been driving down the freeway and passed right by your exit? Or walked into a room and can't remember what you are looking for? Or the best one is finish eating a meal and not even remembering eating those last few bites? During those moments, you were living in your head and not in real life.

So often our brains are on overdrive and we are thinking about the next task on our list, that last conversation, or what's for dinner. A friend of mine gave me the idea of thinking, "be here now" a gentle reminder to get out of your head and into your life.

Imagine how many precious moments you could enjoy more fully by being present. Imagine what you can learn from conversations if you are not thinking about what you are going to say next, but genuinely listening to your friend or child. Imagine how much joy you would experience in the simple things by actually feeling them. Things like:

- The hot water in the shower
- The delicious food on your dinner plate
- The warm hug from your spouse
- The exciting story from your child

Do you ever go through your day half listening, half living? We are meant to truly experience life and to feel joy, sorrow, frustration, humor, and love.

So often we stuff away our feelings and numb out! What we must do is be present, live fully, and experience the beauty of a life well lived.

Eating mindfully is VERY important. Slowing down, chewing your food until liquid, placing your fork down between bites, and enjoying pleasant conversations are all important practices during meal times.

Slowing down allows your brain signals of satiety to be registered. Oftentimes before the brain says it's had enough, you have eaten too much.

Since digestion begins in your mouth, proper chewing allows the enzymes in your saliva to break down your food, making it easier on your stomach and small intestine to complete the digestion process. This also frees up energy to be used in other areas of your body!

Life passes by fast enough. Slow down, be present and live fully!

CHALLENGE – Take 2 pieces of chocolate. (Please don't read this until you actually have 2 pieces of chocolate to fully do this experiment.)

Now place one in your mouth and eat it as you would normally. Do it now…. skip the rest of this text until you actually eat that chocolate!

Next place the second one in your mouth and simply let it melt. Do not chew or bite down. Savor the silky experience. Record your feelings and notice which method you prefer.

I learned this at a Geneen Roth seminar and found it very interesting to notice which method I preferred. Savoring the finer things in life is such a rich experience.

FEED YOURSELF: FERMENTED FOODS

Growing up, I absolutely hated sauerkraut. My mom used to make me eat it with smoked kielbasa and it gagged me every time. That was the canned stuff of course.

Fast forward 45 years and now I make it from scratch. I love eating it with grass-fed kielbasa, mustard, and jalapenos.

Gut health is all the rage these days and a very important aspect in the overall health of our body.

Fermented foods feed the gut by adding healthy bacteria. And the lactic acid, produced during fermentation, helps the healthy bacteria proliferate. Since our immune system resides in our gut, eating these delicious foods will help boost your immunity.

The most popular fermented food is sauerkraut. But there is also kimchi, dill pickles (made without vinegar), kefir, yogurt, and kombucha.

Fermented foods aid digestion because the bacteria predigests. It is a great practice to have a couple of bites of fermented foods at the beginning of each meal.

Fermented foods contain up to 10 trillion probiotic organisms. You can get more probiotics from fermented foods than from a probiotic supplement.

By regulating your microbiome and also helping your taste buds adjust to a more bitter/sour flavor, this may help reduce sugar cravings.

Every month, I brew a batch of Kombucha and take a couple sips every day. Talk about looking nasty, if you have ever seen a batch of kombucha brewing, you know what I am talking about!

It's the scoby on top that looks disgusting, but it is just a Symbiotic Culture of Bacteria and Yeast.

Kombucha is fermented tea. Simply put, it's a batch of sweet tea with a scoby on top that eats the sugar to create a fermented beverage. The flavor is a bit tangy, a bit sweet, and mildly fizzy. Kind of like a healthy soda!

You can purchase kombucha in the grocery store in the refrigerated section. I love the Cherry and Chia Seed flavor as it has an interesting mouth feel!

"It is shown that kombucha can efficiently act in health preservation and recovery due to four main properties: detoxification, anti-oxidation, energizing potencies, and promotion of boosting immunity." Dr. Josh Axe [56]

He also states that it helps with joint health and weight loss.

Please know that I didn't like it the first time I tried it But, after realizing all the amazing health benefits, I forced myself to keep drinking it. My favorite way is to cut it with sparkling water...then it's less sweet!

Homemade Kombucha

Boil 2 quarts of water, 8 black tea bags, and 1 cup sugar for 10 minutes. Fill a one-gallon mason jar with cooled tea. Place scoby on top of tea. Cover jar with paper towel and write date on it. Secure with rubber band and place in pantry (covered with towel) for 15-20 days.

Be careful to not touch scoby with metal or plastic. Test mixture with wooden spoon. The longer the tea brews the less sweet and the more sparkly.

Pour in bottles and either place in pantry, to continue the fermentation, or refrigerate.

You can purchase dehydrated SCOBYs online.

Simple Fermented Sauerkraut

1 head of Cabbage
2 T Sea Salt

Cut cabbage in quarters. Thinly slice each quarter and sprinkle with salt. Knead the cabbage for about 10 minutes. Liquid will begin to collect.

Place cabbage in a jar or fermentation vessel and pour liquid brine over the top. If needed, add water until cabbage is complete submerged.

Fill a baggie with water and stuff into top of jar to fill any air space. Cover with a cloth and rubber band.

Place in pantry and check flavor after about 2 weeks. Depending on temperature, it may take up to 5 weeks to get to desired flavor.

To create more oxytocin in your life:Laugh, play, hug, look into someone's eyes and smile, give gratitude and thanks, play with a pet, and stay in the present (so difficult for many of us). So yes, you can hug that belly fat away! Learn to control the stress you can (and learn to manage your thoughts around the stress you simply can't control). Remember, stress is a normal and actually a healthy part of life when we have perceived control around it and internal peace within it. Make a proactive effort to carve out time in each day to connect with others (an easy one? Don't eat watching the TV!)"[57]

~ Dr. Anna Cabeca

Day 14 Love Yourself: Date Night

A Date night can be with your spouse, your child, a friend, or even yourself. It is a time to take a break, unplug from social media, and enjoy the simple things.

When my kids were younger, I used to take them on a simple date once a month, around the time of their birthdate. My first son was born on Dec 1st. So, on or around the 1st of every month, we would go on a simple date. This may be to get an ice cream, to the movie, park or to lunch. Now granted, I wish this were a practice I had started MUCH earlier in their lives and continued much later.

Now for the juicy part! Many of my "date nights" are home dates (my husband's choice). We love when the house is empty and we can chill out by the pool, have some wine or margaritas, and relax.

My favorite date night is dinner out and a movie. I really like the movie first and then go to dinner so we can talk about the movie.

The best rule is: NO PHONES, unless to take a selfie together!

Take time and talk about the highlights of the week, the dreams you have for your future, the love you feel for others, and the passion that drives you each day. And then, skip dessert and head home for the real icing on the cake: SEX!

Yep, it's part of what we are created to do. So many great hormones, especially oxytocin, are released in your body and will benefit your health journey.

Oftentimes we are too busy and let sex become an unimportant part of our life (unless you are a man and it's #1 on your list). Honestly, I always think God has a sense of humor. Most women I know, don't even have it on their list, and for their men it's always #1.

We must realize how important it really is...making our partner happy, filling our body with endorphins (feel good hormones), and bonding as a couple.

CHALLENGE: Schedule a date night this weekend. Make it very special and journal about your experience.

FEED YOURSELF: FAT BURNING SPICES

Seasoning your food not only adds flavor, but many also have health benefits. These are my top three spices for a variety of reasons.

Cayenne provides the spicy flavor I love in my food and it also boosts the metabolism. My hubby sweats when he eats those hot chili peppers, so you know it must be working! It's the capsaicin in peppers that also helps with digestion and kidney function.

Cinnamon not only adds a great flavor, but it also helps stabilize blood sugar, boosts brain function, and increases energy [58].... Plus, it is a prebiotic which fertilizes the gut microbiome.

Turmeric, aka curcumin, is a natural anti-inflammatory and antioxidant. I add it to my smoothies to help with inflammation in my knees

Researcher Bharat Aggarwal is bullish on curcumin's potential as a cancer treatment, particularly in colon, prostate and breast cancers; preliminary studies have found that curcumin can inhibit tumor cell growth and suppress enzymes that activate carcinogens.[59]

Ways to Enjoy:

Cayenne: Tacos, lemon water,
Cinnamon: smoothies, coffee,
Turmeric: butter chicken, tikka masala

Golden Milk

1 can Coconut Milk
1 tsp Turmeric
1 tsp Cinnamon
1 tsp ground Cardamom
1 tsp ground Ginger
1 pinch of Black Pepper
1 dropper Stevia

Place all ingredients in blender. Blend until smooth. Heat on stove.
Pour into 2 mugs and sip slowly.

"Cinnamon helps level blood sugar and reduce the insulin spike in the human body. This allows the body to remain more sensitive to carbohydrates in a good way (muscle growth and fat loss) but more importantly can help prevent a nasty blood sugar crash halfway through the day"[60]

~ Thomas DeLauer

DAY 15 LOVE YOURSELF: ORGANIZE YOUR LIFE

Fail to plan and plan to fail. Do you wing it each day or is your schedule planned out? Instead of being scattered, it's best to be organized. Not just with your calendar, but with your fitness, meals, drawers, cupboards, closets, garage, and everything else.

When your home or work life is in disarray it spreads to other areas of your life. This was one of my biggest struggles.

My house is kept fairly clean, other than the usual mess with 3 boys and 2 dogs. But I tend to take on way too much. There are just so many awesome things to do, right? All of my projects have tended to be spread out on the kitchen table. With the help of binders and filing folders, this is no longer a problem.

When you look at the overall task of getting organized, here are some words of wisdom.

A. Write a list of ALL the things you need to get done in your home environment. List everything big and small. Then set aside a whole day, from waking up until bed time and knock as many items off the list as you can. This means no TV, phone calls, Facebook, or any other distractions. Just get'er done cowgirl.

B. Another method is taking that same list and doing one thing every day for an entire week or month or however long it takes. Set a goal date of when it must be complete.

Winter is such a great time to do this, since you won't be tempted as much to go outside and play!

For daily organization... I like doing a Set-up Sunday!

This means that I plan my dinners, make the grocery list and shop for what I need for the week. I plan my workout schedule, and the big projects I need to do for work.

Everything else needs to fit in the nooks and crannies. Since I am a Free Spirit by nature, I love having those pockets of time where I can sub at the gym, meet a friend for lunch, or have a last-minute pedicure!

Which do you choose? Suggestion A, B, or both? By both, I mean start with A and then finish the list with B. That's my favorite option!

FEED YOURSELF: HEMP SEED

I always thought this was a bad thing – kind of like pot or weed. Only when I took the time to learn about the health benefits did I start eating this seed on my salads and yogurt.

Hemp seeds are rich in healthy fats! Hemp hearts are over 30% fat and contain great fatty acids, particularly omega 3 and omega 6. Hemp also contains GLA, which is harder to find and prevents inflammation. GLA also helps to bind and balance the body's hormones. [61]

Since they contain high amounts of the amino acid L-arginine, which produces nitric oxide, they may lower blood pressure and reduce the risk of heart disease. Since heart disease is the #1 killer of men and women, I think a little hemp seed is a good addition to your diet. Don't you?

Hemp seeds are rich in amino acids and are a complete source of protein. 25% of the calories in hemp seeds actually come from protein. Hemp seeds have a great amount of soluble fiber and insoluble fiber, which benefits our digestive health and helps us enjoy a healthy poop. So fear not my little angel and add some hemp seeds to your daily routine.

Hot Hemp Cereal

½ cup hulled Hemp Seeds
1 T Coconut Flour
1 cup Coconut Milk
Dash of Salt
1 dropper of Liquid Stevia

Mix all ingredients and cook on med/low heat until thick. You can top with a pat of butter or some sliced berries and cinnamon.

Hemp Pilaf

1 cup Hemp Seeds
2 T Olive Oil or Butter
1 cup Sliced Mushrooms
¼ cup Sliced Almonds
½ cup Chicken Broth
1 T chopped Parsley
½ tsp Garlic Powder
Salt and Pepper

Sauté mushrooms in olive oil or butter. When mushrooms are soft, add hemp seeds, and mix well. Add broth and seasonings. Simmer on medium-low until broth is absorbed. Top with almonds and serve.

DAY 16 LOVE YOURSELF: LAUGH

One of my favorite things to do is laugh; a good deep belly laugh is so fun. The last good one I had was when my son was making fun of my cooking.

Many of my best laughs are laughing at myself. Stop taking life so seriously...laughing at our own stupidity can be fun!

Laughing literally relieves stress, lowers blood pressure, decreases inflammation, improves memory, and shuts down the stress hormone cortisol (which leads to belly fat storage). Wonder if we can laugh ourselves thin?[62]

Laughing at a movie or while out with family and friends is my favorite. Sometimes I like watching stupid movies just to get a good laugh.... and there is something about being in a theater with other people laughing, that makes the experience better.

I cannot stand that fake canned laughter on sitcoms though. Not sure why, but it bugs the crap out of me. Except of course Seinfeld and Friends (am I showing my age?)

Some of my favorite funny movies are

- Bridesmaids
- Wedding Crashers
- Meet the Parents
- Notting Hill
- When Harry Met Sally
- Old School
- Shrek
- Elf
- Airplane!
- Foul Play

YouTube is another great resource to find funny videos; your friends are probably posting them to Facebook daily. Many of these crazy videos are of people taping their babies, puppies or cats and are quite hilarious!

CHALLENGE: Find something and laugh out loud at the very least once a day.

FEED YOURSELF: CHIA SEED

Ch-Ch-Ch-Chia…. you must remember those crazy animals that you spread with black seed, water them, and watch them grow. Who would have ever thought they would later come to the mainstream as a super food?

One tablespoon of Chia seeds has 2.5 grams of Omega 3's that's like gagging down 5 fish oil capsules.

Basic Chia Pudding

2 cups unsweetened Coconut Milk
1 cup Chia Seeds
½ t Vanilla
1 dropper of Liquid Stevia

Shake together and chill for an hour. Shake again and chill for another hour. Shake again. Chill for 2 more hours. Serve in bowls and enjoy!

Peanut Butter Cup Yogurt

2/3 cup unsweetened Almond Milk Yogurt
1 T Chocolate Protein Powder
1 T Chia Seeds
1 T Peanut Butter

Mix chia seeds into yogurt and let set for one hour. Stir in protein powder and peanut butter and enjoy.

Day 17 Love Yourself: Pets

Man's best friend (and woman's) is the dog.

My dogs, Rocky and Ringo, don't yell at me, judge me, gossip about me, ignore me, hurt my feelings, or any of the other thing's women tend to do to each other.

They are always happy to see me, love being petted, and don't care what I am wearing or how loud I am.

Oftentimes, life is lonely, and we need a friend. That's where a pet comes in handy. Dogs, cats, horses, guinea pigs, or even fish can brighten your day!

My favorite thing about having a dog is they make me take them for a walk every day! We have a path near our home that is 2 miles and they love walking out there, especially when the sun is shining or after a rain when there are puddles to play in.

If it's not possible to have a pet of your own, who do you know that has a pet you can visit regularly? Or maybe a neighbor has a dog that needs a walk. How cool would it be for you to help your neighbor and yourself at the same time?

Seniors are one community that definitely benefit from having a pet. When my mom moved into assisted living and had to give up her dog, she was so sad. It broke my heart. I hope she can get a cat to bring her joy.

Feed Yourself: Pastured Chicken

One of my favorite sources of protein is chicken. Most Sundays, I marinate and grill up a bunch of chicken. After it cools down, I simply chop them up and store them in glassware for the week. Then I can throw the chicken on my salad for lunch, which makes meal planning super convenient.

Just like the egg, chicken labeling has different meanings.

- All-Natural – no artificial ingredients
- Farm Raised- aren't they all?
- Raised cage free – still indoors just no cages
- No hormones added – not allowed anyways
- Raised without Antibiotics – as stated
- Rocky and Rosie – Both free-range, without antibiotics, just Rosie eats an organic, GMO free diet.
- Free-Range – are able to go outside (as little as 5 minutes a day)
- Organic – free range, no antibiotics

Chicken is also high in B vitamins and selenium, giving you energy, antioxidant protection and thyroid support.[63]

Chicken Fajitas

1 pound of organic chicken breast
½ cup olive oil
½ cup Bragg's liquid aminos
½ cup Honey
2 Onions, thinly sliced
2 Red Bell Peppers, thinly sliced
2 T Olive Oil
Blend liquids and marinate chicken overnight.

Grill on BBQ for about 15 minutes per side depending on size. Let cool for 10 minutes and slice thin. Sauté onions and bell peppers in 2T olive oil until carmelized. Serve with hot sauce, guacamole, cheese and sour cream

NOTE: Instead of the traditional tortilla, I make a yummy fajita bowl.

Butter Chicken

2 T Butter
1 small Red Onion, chopped
2 T Fresh Garlic, chopped
1 T Fresh Ginger, chopped
2 T Tomato Paste
1 T Stevia
1 T Cumin Seeds
1 T Garam Masala
1 tsp Red Pepper Flakes
1 t Turmeric
1 t Salt
1 lb Boneless Chicken, cubed
½ cup Coconut Milk
¼ cup Water

Heat oil in skillet. Add onion, garlic, and ginger, and cook until golden. Add tomato paste, sugar, cumin, garam masala, red chili flakes, turmeric and salt. Cook for 2 minutes. Add chicken cubes and stir to coat well. Add the yogurt and water and cook about 8 minutes or until chicken is cooked through.

Day 18 Love Yourself: Feel Good Movies and Books

One of my favorite things to do is watch a really happy movie or read a really fun book. Something that you can get so absorbed in, life's troubles seem non-existent, and you can transport yourself into another space.

When we take a mental break and give ourselves light-hearted fun, it's not only enjoyable, but it's restful. Ranker.com posted the Top 10 Books to Make You Feel Good (I am going to have to read more of these)

- Harry Potter
- The Art of Racing in the Rain
- A Prayer for Owen Meany
- The Glass Castle
- The Help
- Wild: From Lost to Found on the Pacific Crest Trail
- Something blue
- Kane and Abel
- The Happiness Project
- To Kill a Mockingbird[64]

And the Top 10 Feel Good Movies

- The Shawshank Redemption
- Mrs. Doubtfire
- Finding Nemo
- Big
- It's a Wonderful Life
- Cool Runnings
- When Harry Met Sally
- The Breakfast Club
- Willy Wonka & the Chocolate Factory
- A League of Their Own[65]

Elf, which is one of my favorites, was #14. I just had to include it here because I just LOVE that movie!

125

CHALLENGE: Watch one of these movies and buy one of these books. Enjoy them so you can relax and quiet your mind before bed.

FEED YOURSELF: SARDINES

When I was a little girl, my Sicilian father would enjoy sardines, smoked oysters, sharp cheddar and Ritz crackers. I would sit with him and enjoy them as well. He would even let me drink about ½ cup of beer with him.

Sardines are rich in omega-3 fatty acids. The reason they are called essential, is because our body cannot produce them, so we must eat them. Omega 3's Fatty Acids are shown to be helpful in preventing heart disease. These healthy fats are also known to break down arterial plaque, which blocks arteries and increases blood pressure.

Smaller than salmon, these sea creatures do not contain as much mercury as the larger fish salmon and tuna. My favorite brand is Wild Planet, and I have tried just about every brand; these just taste less fishy.

Sardines are one of the best sources of calcium and Vitamin D which may prevent certain types of cancer. Sardines are good suppliers of proteins. Proteins are made up of amino acids, which are the essential building blocks of life. The protein that is found in sardines can reduce insulin resistance and build muscles.

They are also high in selenium which has major anti-oxidant benefits. Selenium helps neutralize free radicals and protect the organs from damage.

Sardines are low in calories, which helps with weight-loss, but provides the protein and vitamins we need to maintain a healthy metabolism.

Ways to Enjoy:

Sardine "Sushi"

1 Can of sardines
1 package Nori Squares
Avocado
Chipotle mayo

Wrap sardines in nori, top with avocado and a bit of mayo, fold and eat.

Sardine Snack

1 can Sardines
½ Avocado, sliced
Pork Rinds
Cilantro chopped
1 Lime, cut in four

Place a sardine on a large pork rind. Top with avocado, cilantro and squeeze of lime.

"Sardines (even canned ones) are great because they are one of the few animal foods that we still consume all of it, including the bones and skin. While this makes people squeamish, these "off bits" of the fish have important vitamins and minerals, including a great dose of calcium from the bones. One can contains about 1/3 of the recommended daily amount of calcium in a highly absorbable form."[66]

~Katie Wells, Wellness Mama

Day 19 Love Yourself: Grow a Garden

When my husband drug me out of the city and planted my ass on a farm, I was NOT a happy girl. The flies, snakes, and dust were ridiculous. Then he planted my first garden and I quickly turned from hate to love!

Growing your own food is such a fantastic experience that I would love to see you be able to enjoy this process. Not only does the food taste way better, it is much more nutritious.

There is something about putting your hands in dirt (other than getting dirt under your fingernails) that is healing to your body and your mind. Pulling weeds can actually be relaxing and the Vitamin D you soak in from the sun is the happy vitamin. The minerals soaking into your skin from the soil is healing and enjoying nature's frogs and worms brings you joy!

Last year my hubby planted an amazing garden and I was out there picking strawberries and other veggies. One day this small frog jumped onto my hand and scared the crap out of me.

There are literally health benefits from gardening that go beyond the healthy food.

USA Today reports that Horticulture therapy helps people suffering from addiction recovery and mental health issues, conditions from dementia to eating disorders. "Horticultural therapy stimulates thought, exercises the body and encourages an awareness of the external environment. Moreover, the clients who have benefited from this type of therapy report a renewed desire to live, decreased anxiety and improved self-worth."[67]

So maybe you don't live on a farm and that's ok! Whether you have a big or small yard, there are plenty of ways to build a garden. My parents plant their tomatoes and peppers in big blue tubs on their patio.

No yard at all? No problem, you can have an indoor garden. Now of course you won't get the exact same experience, but at least you will get great tasting, healthy produce!

Shelves are a great space saver. All you need is enough light. You can purchase different lights, depending on the size of your room, and the sunlight you get. Room temps should be at 65-75 degrees.[68] Try it out with herbs. They seem to work well for me!

A Community Garden is another great way to play in the dirt. This is where the city designates a large plot of land and different people get to use a small portion for their own personal use and for a very nominal fee.

Feed Yourself: Coconut Oil

There is a jar of coconut oil in my pantry and a jar in my bathroom. I start the day with 1 tsp of coconut oil in my coffee, use it for cooking, and if I bake, it's a fantastic choice of fat.

In some studies, somewhere in Asia I presume, Sumo wrestlers were given loads of coconut oil in an attempt to fatten them up. What happened? They started losing weight at an alarming rate. This is because coconut oil actually has a thermogenic effect, helping to speed up the body's natural metabolic rate.[69]

Coconut oil is a medium chain triglyceride. Bodybuilders have been adding MCT oil to their diet as an energy source in their typical low carb diets.

It can also:

- Boost HDL (good cholesterol)
- Increase your energy
- Burn Fat
- Kill Bacteria, Viruses, and Infections

Coconut Oil is also great for Oil Pulling. This is an ancient Ayurvedic practice, which will clean your mouth from bacteria, improve gum health, whiten teeth and help prevent bad breath.

Simply take about 1 tablespoon of coconut oil and let it melt in your mouth. Swish it around for about 15-20 minutes. Then spit it out into the garbage and rinse your mouth with fresh water.

My favorite dessert recipe is below and made with coconut oil.

Peanut Butter Balls

½ cup Coconut Oil
½ cup Peanut Butter
2 T Cacao Powder
1 dropper of Liquid Stevia

Place all ingredients in a small pot and heat on low. Mix well. Pour into small candy molds and freeze until firm. Remove from molds and store in glass container in refer.

Day 20 Love Yourself: Stress Soothers

Let's face it girls, we live in Busyland. When we are not busy doing something, we have down time, and we fill it up. Hopefully with something that feeds you.

The top stressors in life are death of a loved one, illness, divorce, financial problems, loss of job, relationship issues and the list goes on. It is pretty much impossible to not experience stress in life.

Have you heard the saying "stress kills"? It is so very true! Stress taxes our bodies in so many ways that we must find means to manage it.

When you experience stress, how do you cope? Do you become frazzled? Do you shut down? Do you overeat? Under eat? We all handle stresses differently and some methods are healthier than others.

Let's brainstorm some methods, which will help you manage stress:

- Take a hot bath with candles
- Go for a walk-in nature
- Play with a child
- Pray or meditate
- Deep breathing exercises
- Meet a friend for coffee
- Do a yoga class
- Workout and sweat it off
- And my favorite – have a great glass of wine!

If you eat to manage your stress, you are essentially stuffing it away. So, while the food may take the stress away for a few minutes; in the long run, it makes things worse because you will feel guilty and disappointed in yourself.

Just remember: Nothing tastes as good as healthy feels

CHALLENGE: Practice the above stress management methods and journal about your experiences.

FEED YOURSELF: BERRIES

Last summer my hubby planted about 80' of strawberries and we enjoyed them fresh all summer long. We also froze a bunch to enjoy in our smoothies.

Berries are very low in calories, have a low glycemic index, and are high in fiber. They are simply the best choice among fruits in my humble opinion.

While Blueberries are considered a super food, all berries have health benefits including reduced risk of:

- Heart Disease
- Stroke
- Cancer
- Blood Pressure
- Diabetes
- Depression[70]

Since strawberries are a high pesticide crop, and on the list of the Dirty Dozen, please purchase organic whenever possible.

Be careful not to overeat berries. They are best as a topping on yogurt or a salad, instead of eating by the handful. Even though they are the healthiest fruit, they do have sugar.

Ways to enjoy:

- Add to a Smoothie
- Top Greek Yogurt
- Snack on Frozen Berries

Spinach Strawberry Salad

2 cups Baby Spinach
½ cup Strawberries, sliced
¼ cup Crumbled Feta Cheese
2 slices of Red Onion
¼ cup Walnuts
1 T Balsamic Vinegar
2 T Extra Virgin Olive Oil

Fill large bowl with baby spinach. Top with strawberries, onion, cheese and walnuts. Drizzle with balsamic vinegar, oil, sea salt and black pepper. For a complete meal, top this salad with chicken breast slices.

Chocolate Dipped Strawberries

1 cup Lily's chocolate chips
1T Coconut Oil
32 Strawberries

Melt chips and oil together. Mix Well. Holding the green side of the strawberry, dip in chocolate and set on wax paper to dry.

"What if I fall?

Oh, but darling, what if you fly?" [71]

~Erin Hanson

DAY 21 LOVE YOURSELF: MASSAGE

Splendid Feet is one of my favorite places to visit on the weekends. For $25 you get a full hour of relaxation through Chinese Reflexology. When I first visited this place, I had no idea what a treat I was in for.

Imagine a large room filled with oversized reclining chairs, soft music, and lovely silent videos of nature on a big screen (and the dude snoring off in la la land next to me, oh wait, that's my hubby)

This is a place where you can get a relaxing massage, with your clothes on, for a great price and get health benefits through pressure points in your feet.

In reflexology, there are locations on the bottom of your feet that correspond to an organ in your body. By applying pressure to the spot, some sort of magic release takes place.

Traditional massage is another wonderful option. You can choose Swedish, deep tissue, sports massage, shiatsu, and others. I love the Gestalt technique taught at Esalen, in Big Sur. My hubby and I really want to do a couple's massage class there someday.

There are many health benefits of massage including:

- improves sleep
- releases toxins
- relieves back pain
- boosts immunity
- counters depression
- reduces stress
- and just feels so damn good!

Sometimes when we have a quiet house, which is very infrequent, my hubby lays out blankets in front of the fire. He heats some oil, turns on soft music, and pours wine so we can trade massages. It is one of his favorite things to do and in writing this, we may have to give the kids money for a movie this weekend!

Self-Massage is another great technique for relaxation. You can use a foam roller, Thera Cane, scalp head massager (yummy), a muscle roller stick, or even those crazy things you can sit on in your car.

Feed Yourself: Aloe Vera

Aloe Vera has been used in wellness for 5,000 years. It's a really good plant to keep in your kitchen in case of burns. Drinking the juice is shown to have:

- Digestive Benefits: ulcers, IBS, colitis, boosts healthy bacteria
- Immunity Benefits: anti-bacterial, anti-viral, anti-fungal
- Heart benefits: lower cholesterol, reduce fatty deposits and blood clots in arteries.[72]

Aloe Vera Juice has become so popular you can find it at many health focused stores, such as Sprouts and Vitamin Shoppe.

All you have to do is drink 4-8 ounces every evening before bed.

Bonus Day Love Yourself: Passionate Purpose

Boredom is a common reason why depression may creep in and people may overeat. This is also a time when negative thoughts float through your head. However, if you spend your time and energy focusing on a special project, creating a passion and a purpose, the days fly by and the excitement in life builds.

Often, as we grow older, we forget to dream. Ask yourself what do you love to do? Discover your purpose by brainstorming and making a list of all your favorite things. Set a timer for 15 minutes and mindlessly get that list going. Afterwards, start crossing things off your list until you come up with your top three to five. When I did this, mine were writing a book, teaching fitness classes, being a motivational speaker, and providing nutrition education workshops.

Last year, I did a class with Natasha Hazlett called Unstoppable Influencer, and she made me realize that we are all born with gifts and the world deserves to see them, That means all of us girl!

My passion is helping women to age stronger, to stop the dieting/bingeing roller coaster and nourish themselves. I could not wait to wake up in the morning and finish writing this book, or making a new video, or interviewing a guest for my podcast. I live on purpose.

CHALLENGE: If money and time weren't an issue, what would you be doing? Start discovering your passionate purpose right now!

> "Are you living by purpose, or are you living by default?"
>
> ~Natasha Hazlett

FEED YOURSELF: DARK CHOCOLATE AND RED WINE

Saving the best for last ...dark chocolate and red wine are considered healthy treats.

Dark chocolate is high in fiber, minerals, antioxidants, may lower blood pressure, raise good cholesterol, lower risk of heart disease, improve brain function, and protect your skin against the sun.

My favorite brand is Lily's as it is sweetened with stevia, instead of sugar. Now don't go pigging out on it or anything. But remember in a previous chapter, occasionally let a small piece melt on your tongue and experience that silky enjoyment.

When you buy dark chocolate, look for the highest percent of cocoa you can get, at least 70%. The higher the percentage, the less sugar.[73]

Living in wine country, I do my fair share of drinking red wine (occasionally a buttery white as well).

Red wine has been touted to lower the risk of coronary heart disease. And since this is the number one killer of both men and women, it seems pretty important.

"The lowest risk was seen among women who drank one to two drinks per day on five to six days per week."[74]

Now if you don't currently drink alcohol, I would not recommend starting simply because of this. However, moderation is the key, and it just might help you!

Health Magazine said," Resveratrol, the famed antioxidant found in grape skin, stops fat storage. Studies show that moderate wine drinkers have narrower waists and less belly fat than liquor drinkers."[75]

Your reward day is the perfect time to relax and slow down with a glass of nitrate free red wine and a piece of dark chocolate. The two pair quite nicely for that extra special treat.

Practice Daily

So now you have enjoyed 21 days of loving yourself with important self-care and feeding yourself some of the most nutritious foods on the planet.

Print up the checklist on the book bonus page at my website: www.highenergygirl.com/nfwbonus

Everyday circle each practice you enjoyed as you love and feed yourself. The more circles you can squeeze in to your day, the more you will be crowding out the crap and loving yourself to health!

Don't forget to move your body every day! Learn to love exercise and enjoy the endorphin kick it will bring to your day. Don't tell me you are too tired because the more you move, the more energy you will enjoy!

Increase your energy, empower your life!

Join my Transformation and learn how to be strong in your mind and in your body! The more you practice self-care, the faster you are on your way to more energy, getting fit, and releasing all those unwanted pounds.

XO Cheers to Your Health! *Tracie*

> I want
> to inspire people.
> I want
> someone to look
> at me and say
> "Because of you, I did not give up."

THE HIGH ENERGY GIRL MANIFESTO

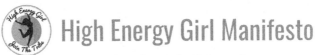

High Energy Girl Manifesto

MEET THE NEW YOU!

TIME TO GET SERIOUS, *Feel Sexy and Alive*, **STRONG** AND VIBRANT.
DRAW A ~~LINE~~ IN THE SAND AND **COMMIT** TO LIVING YOUR **BEST** *Life*!
NO STARTING MONDAY, **NO** WHINING AND **NO** MORE EXCUSES.

YOU DESERVE TO BE THE **BEST YOU** POSSIBLE, INSPIRE OTHERS AND *Feel Younger*!
IT'S NEVER **TOO LATE, TO LIVE THE LIFE YOU DREAM ABOUT,** IN
THE BODY YOU DESERVE!

TO FEEL *High Energy* ALL DAY, EVERYDAY!
YOU MAY BE A LADY, BUT YOU FEEL LIKE A GIRL!

A HIGH ENERGY GIRL	is **strong** and **empowered**, builds herself up, so she can build up others. Competes only with herself and **focuses** on the weights in the gym going up, rather than the weight on the scale going down.
A HIGH ENERGY GIRL	eats healthy food to fuel her body because she wants to **heal** and be strong. She is *intuitive* and knows exactly what she needs. Sometimes it's a friend, sometimes it's a walk or a hot bath, sometimes it's a steak or a nice glass of wine.
A HIGH ENERGY GIRL	*Loves* herself completely, without judgement, and treats herself as she would treat a newborn baby. She nourishes her soul with compassion, joy, love, and forgiveness.
A HIGH ENERGY GIRL	has *integrity* and keeps all the promises she makes to herself and to others. She **values** her community and loves to serve and help people who need it.

TAKE THE PLEDGE AND BEGIN TODAY!

You are a High Energy Girl Now!

Start Your Journey at HighEnergyTransformation.com

End Notes

1. "Family Cancer Syndromes." American Cancer Society. Accessed May 19, 2019. https://www.cancer.org/cancer/cancer-causes/genetics/family-cancer-syndromes.html

2. Taubes, Gary. "What's Cholesterol Got to Do With It?" The New York Times. January 27, 2008. Accessed May 19, 2019. https://www.nytimes.com/2008/01/27/opinion/27taubes.html.

3. Pollan, Michael. *The Omnivore's Dilemma.* Penguin, 2007.

4. Dove, Laurie L. "Top 10 Groceries Americans Buy - HowStuffWorks." *HowStuffWorks.* InfoSpace LLC, n.d. Web. 03 Dec. 2014.

5. Hyman, Mark, M.D. "5 Reasons High Fructose Corn Syrup Will Kill You - Dr. Mark Hyman." *Dr. Mark Hyman.* N.p., 18 Oct. 2014. Web. 01 Dec. 2014.

6. Singleton, Bonnie. "Why Is Phosphoric Acid Bad for You?" *LIVESTRONG.COM.* Demand Media, Inc., 21 Oct. 2013. Web. 02 Dec. 2014.

7 Culliney, Kacey. "Cereal Blockbusters: America's Top 10 Best-Selling Brands." *BakeryAndSnacks.com.* William Reed Business Media, 22 July 2013. Web. 03 Dec. 2014.

8. Michaëlsson, Karl, Alicja Wolk, Sophie Langenskiöld, Samar Basu, Eva Warensjö Lemming, Håkan Melhus, and Liisa Byberg. "Milk Intake and Risk of Mortality and Fractures in Women and Men." *Thebmj.* The BMJ, 22 Sept. 2014. Web. 03 Dec. 2014.

9. Atkinson, Fiona S., Kaye Foster-Powell, and Jennie C. Brand-Miller. "Glycemic Index and Glycemic Load for 100+ Foods." *Glycemic Index and Glycemic Load for 100+ Foods.* Harvard University, n.d. Web. 01 Dec. 2014.

End Notes

10. Mercola, Joseph, M.D. "Processed Foods Lead to Cancer and Early Death – Dr. Joseph Mercola". *Dr. Joseph Mercola*. n.d., 27 Feb. 2019. Web. 13 May 2019

11. Strauss, Valerie. "Rats Find Oreos as Addictive as Cocaine." *Washington Post.* The Washington Post, 18 Oct. 2013. Web. 03 Dec. 2014.

12. Gunnars, Kris. "10 Disturbing Reasons Why Sugar Is Bad For You." *Authority Nutrition.* Authority Nutrition, n.d. Web. 02 Dec. 2014.

13. Hyman, Mark, M.D. "How Diet Soda Makes You Fat (and Other Food and Diet Industry Secrets) - Dr. Mark Hyman." *Dr. Mark Hyman.* n.d., 22 Feb. 2013. Web. 03 Dec. 2014.

14. "How & Why To Feel Your Feelings." Christie Inge. July 12, 2018. Accessed May 19, 2019. https://christieinge.com/feel-your-feelings/.

15. "What Is Stress? Symptoms, Signs & More." Cleveland Clinic. Accessed May 19, 2019. https://my.clevelandclinic.org/health/articles/11874-stress.

16. Goldberg, Joseph, M.D. "The Effects of Stress on Your Body." *WebMD.* WebMD, 24 June 2014. Web. 03 Dec. 2014.

17. Phillips, Bill, and Michael DOrso. *Body for Life 12 Weeks to Mental and Physical Strength.* New York: HarperCollins, 1999.

18. Skelly, Samantha. *Hungry for Happiness: One Womans Journey from Fighting Food to Finding Freedom.* United States: Create Space, an Amazon Company, 2017.

19. Rosenthal, Joshua. *Integrative Nutrition: Feed Your Hunger for Health and Happiness.* New York, NY: Integrative Nutrition Pub., 2008. Print.

20 Rosenthal, Joshua. *Integrative Nutrition: Feed Your Hunger for Health and Happiness.* New York, NY: Integrative Nutrition Pub., 2008. Print.

21. Steinberg, Dori M., Deborah F. Tate, Gary G. Bennett, Susan Ennett, Carmen Samuel-Hodge, and Dianne S. Ward. "Abstract." *National Center for Biotechnology Information.* U.S. National Library of Medicine, 02 July 2013. Web.

22. "A Quote by Henry Ford." Goodreads. Accessed May 19, 2019. https://www.goodreads.com/quotes/978-whether-you-think-you-can-or-you-think-you-can-t--you-re.

23. Hyams, Joe. *Zen in the Martial Arts.* New York: Bantam, 1997.

24 Roizen, Michael F. *You: The Owners Manual: An Insiders Guide to the Body That Will Make You Healthier and Younger.* New York, NY: Collins, 2008.

25. Fung, Jason, and Jason Fung. "A New Therapeutic Option for Weight Loss." Medium. July 11, 2018. Accessed May 19, 2019. https://medium.com/@drjasonfung/a-new-therapeutic-option-for-weight-loss-2dc06b72de99.

26. "The Ghost of Your Potential [Les Brown]." YouTube. September 04, 2009. Accessed May 19, 2019. https://youtu.be/bp6bSM6gb4A.

27 "Vision Board Ideas & How to Make Yours Better | Jack Canfield." America's Leading Authority On Creating Success And Personal Fulfillment - Jack Canfield. January 02, 2019. Accessed May 19, 2019. https://www.jackcanfield.com/blog/how-to-create-an-empowering-vision-book/.

28. "18 Benefits of Deep Breathing and How to Breathe Deeply?" *One Powerful Word.* OnePowerfulWord, n.d. Web.

29. Bjarnadottir, Adda, MS. "Coffee and Antioxidants: Everything You Need to Know." Healthline. February 20, 2019. Accessed May 19, 2019. https://www.healthline.com/nutrition/coffee-worlds-biggest-source-of-antioxidants.

End Notes

30. "The Benefits of Coffee: What Your Brain Does on Caffeine." Bulletproof. April 13, 2017. Accessed May 19, 2019. https://blog.bulletproof.com/the-benefits-of-coffee-your-brain-on-caffeine/.

31. Klein, Sarah. "8 Scary Side Effects of Sleep Deprivation." *The Huffington Post.* TheHuffingtonPost.com, 18 Sept. 2014. Web.

32. Emmerich, Maria, and Craig Emmerich. *Keto. the Complete Guide to Success on the Ketogenic Diet, including Simplified Science and No-cook Meal Plans.* Las Vegas, NV: Victory Belt Publishing, 2018.

33. Mares, Nicholas. "Why Our Bone Broth?" Kettle & Fire. Accessed May 19, 2019. https://www.kettleandfire.com/pages/why-our-bone-broth.

34. *About Epsom Salts (MgSO 4 ·7H 2 O)* (n.d.): n. pag. *Epsomsaltcouncil.org.* Universal Health Institute. Web.

35. Murphy, PJ, and SS Campbell. "Nighttime Drop in Body Temperature: A Physiological Trigger for Sleep Onset?" *National Center for Biotechnology Information.* U.S. National Library of Medicine, 20 July 1997. Web.

32. Walding, Brenda, DPT, FDN-P. "Try This One Awesome Cure for Constipation and Immunity Boost." Paleo F(x)™. March 15, 2019. Accessed May 19, 2019. https://www.paleofx.com/cure-constipation/

37. Sutherland, Matt. "Screwing Cancer the Metabolic Way: Meet Dr. Nasha Winters." Foreword Reviews: Book Reviews and Coverage of Indie Publishers. January 08, 2018. Accessed May 19, 2019. https://www.forewordreviews.com/articles/article/screwing-cancer-the-metabolic-way-meet-dr-nasha-winters/.

38. Davis, Bruce, Ph.D. "There Are 50,000 Thoughts Standing Between You and Your Partner Every Day!" *The Huffington Post.* TheHuffingtonPost.com, Inc., 23 May 2013. Web. 03 Dec. 2014.

39. "Polyphenols: Do They Play a Role in the Prevention of Human Pathologies?" *National Center for Biotechnology Information.* U.S. National Library of Medicine, June 2002. Web. 03 Dec. 2014.

40. "EWG's 2014 Shopper's Guide to Pesticides in Produce." *Environmental Working Group.* Environmental Working Group, n.d. Web.

41. Ericson, John. "75% of Americans May Suffer From Chronic Dehydration, According to Doctors." *Medical Daily.* IBT Media Inc., 3 July 2013. Web. 03 Dec. 2014.

42. Zelman, Kathleen M. "Why Drink More Water? See 6 Health Benefits of Water." *WebMD.* WebMD, LLC., n.d. Web. 30 Nov. 2014.

43 "16 Health Benefits of Drinking Warm Lemon Water." *Food Matters.* Permacology Productions Pty Ltd, 2 Jan. 2013. Web. 03 Dec. 2014.

44. Tomovich Jacobsen, Maryann. "Benefits of Fish Oil, Salmon, Walnuts, & More." *WebMD.* WebMD, 09 May 2014. Web. 03 Dec. 2014.

45. Goldfarb, Todd. "Meditation for Beginners: 20 Practical Tips for Quieting the Mind." *Zenhabits.net.* N.p., 7 Nov. 2007. Web. 03 Dec. 2014.

46. Edwards, Rebekah. "One of Nature's Top Cancer-Fighting Foods." Dr. Axe. January 16, 2018. Accessed May 19, 2019. https://draxe.com/broccoli-sprouts/.

47. Wei, Ou Wen. "Overview." Pangu Shengong. Accessed May 19, 2019. http://www.pangu.org/pangu-shengong/overview/.

48. "Avocado Nutrition Facts and Health Benefits." *California Avocado.* California Avocado Commission, n.d. Web.

49. Economy, Peter. "37 Earl Nightingale Quotes That Will Empower You to Soar High." Inc.com. October 02, 2015. Accessed May 19, 2019. https://www.inc.com/peter-economy/37-earl-nightingale-quotes-that-will-empower-you-to-soar-high.html.

50. Jockers, David, DNM, DC, MS. "6 Health Benefits of Grass-Fed Butter." DrJockers.com. January 27, 2018. Accessed May 19, 2019. https://drjockers.com/6-health-benefits-grass-fed-butter/.

51. Nordqvist, Joseph. "What Are the Health Benefits of Almonds?" *Medical News Today*. MediLexicon International, 30 Aug. 2014. Web.

52. Renee, Janet. "How Many Almonds Is 100 Calories?" *LIVESTRONG.COM*. LIVESTRONG.COM, 16 Jan. 2014. Web.

53. "7 Surprising Ways to Use Apple Cider Vinegar." *The Dr. Oz Show*. Harpo Inc., 15 July 2014. Web.

54. "Bragg Apple Cider Vinegar." *Bragg Live Foods*. Bragg, n.d. Web.

55. "Love Your Liver Mod Formula." *AlkalineHealth.net*. Alkaline Health, n.d. Web.

56. "7 Reasons to Drink Kombucha Everyday." *DrAxe.com*. DrAxe.com, n.d. Web.

57. Cabeca, Anna. "Put More Oxytocin into Your Life for a Healthier You." Dr. Anna Cabeca. Accessed May 19, 2019. https://drannacabeca.com/blogs/hormone-imbalance/put-more-oxytocin-into-your-life-for-a-healthier-you.

58. Manitsas, Andrea. "11 Health Benefits of Cinnamon You Need to Know." *Organic Authority*. Organic Authority LLC, 29 Nov. 2010. Web.

59. Hendley, Joyce. "8 of the World's Healthiest Spices." *Eating Well*. Meredith Corporation, Nov.-Dec. 2010. Web.

60. DeLauer, Thomas. "Cinnamon for Weight Loss and Brain Function- Thomas DeLauer." YouTube. November 28, 2015.

Accessed   May   19,   2019.
https://www.youtube.com/watch?v=AmgTfWQkiL4.

61. Hemp, Evo. "9 Nutritional Benefits of Hemp Seeds." Evo Hemp.
July   27,   2018.   Accessed   May   19,   2019.
https://evohemp.com/blogs/hempweek/9-nutritional-benefits-of-
hemp-seeds.

62. Reid, Markham. "Does Laughing Have Real Health Benefits?" *Time*.
Time, 19 Nov. 2014. Web.

63. "Selenium." *The World's Healthiest Foods*. The George Mateljan
Foundation, n.d. Web.

64. "Top 10 Books to Make You Feel Good." *Ranker*. Ranker, n.d. Web.
11 Dec. 2014.

65. "The Best Feel Good Movies." *Ranker*. Ranker, n.d. Web.

66. Wells, Katie. "8 Reasons to Eat Sardines (& How to Make Them
Tasty) | Wellness Mama." Wellness Mama®. January 23, 2019.
Accessed   May   19,   2019.
https://wellnessmama.com/252465/sardines-benefits/.

67. Savacool, Julia. "Health Benefits Bloom by Digging in the Garden."
USA Today. Gannett, 11 May 2014. Web.

68. Vinje, Eric. "How to Garden Indoors." *Planet Natural*. Planet Natural
RSS, n.d. Web.

69. Goodman, Alexandra. "Fats and Oils." *Fluid Elevation*. Fluid
Elevation, 2010. Web.

70. Ware, Megan. "What Are the Health Benefits of Strawberries?"
Medical News Today. MediLexicon International, 5 Sept. 2014. Web.

71. Hanson, Erin. "Erin Hanson Quotes (Author of Reverie)."
Goodreads.   Accessed   May   19,   2019.
https://www.goodreads.com/author/quotes/7802403.Erin_Hanson.

End Notes

72. Haris, Nadia. "Health Risks & Benefits of Taking Aloe Vera Juice Internally." *Healthy Eating*. Demand Media, n.d. Web.

73. Gunnars, Kris. "7 Proven Health Benefits of Dark Chocolate." *Authority Nutrition*. Authority Nutrition, n.d. Web

74. Hankinson, Susan E., R.N., Sc.D., Graham A. Colditz, M.D., JoAnn E. Manson, M.D., and Frank E. Speizer, M.D. "Chapter 20: Alcohol." *Healthy Women, Healthy Lives: A Guide to Preventing Disease, from the Landmark Nurses*. Cambridge, MA: Harvard Health Publications, n.d. N. pag. Print.

75. Klein, Sarah. "Best Superfoods for Weight Loss." *Health*. Health Media Ventures Inc., n.d. Web.

JOIN THE TRIBE

Thank you for reading my book. It was very fun to write and I sure hope you plan on being part of the ditch the diet movement.

Head on over to HighEnergyGirl.com and subscribe to my list to be up to date on all podcasts and blog posts. Plus you can get my next book for free at the beginning of the launch.

Don't forget to grab the free bonuses at HighEnergyGirl.com/nfwbonus

Lastly, join my Facebook group: High Energy Girls, where you can ask me anything.

I am always here to help you age stronger and feel younger. You are not too old and it's never to late to get fit, feel sexy and be amazing

Made in the USA
Middletown, DE
12 October 2020

21660128R00089